**"Are you asking me on a date, Lena?"** The confusion on his face had cleared and in its place sat a self-satisfied smirk.

And there it was.

That unbearable arrogance that all the surgeons she'd ever met possessed.

Was it issued to them along with their medical licenses?

"Ugh!" Her hands flew up in irritation. "Why did I ever entertain this idea?"

Annoyance flashed through her, white-hot and simmering on the cusp of anger. Dexter Henry frustrated her more than anyone had in a long time.

"Because you know we'd be perfectly suited to take care of each other's needs." Not a question. There was an undercurrent to his words that took that phrase from simple statement to sensual promise. His gaze moved over her body before he made eye contact once more, making her 1,000 percent certain that he'd meant his words to have multiple meanings.

Her skin heated under the scrutiny of his gaze and she swallowed hard.

She couldn't do this.

"This is a bad idea."

*Or a very good one…*

Dear Reader,

One of the best things about writing romance is that I get to experience the fun of falling in love over and over. With each new couple comes new obstacles, new heartbreaks and the tendrils of fresh new love.

Both distrustful of love, Dex and Lena find themselves in need of dates for holiday events, so they agree to help each other out for the holidays by pretending to be in a relationship. There's a lot at stake—embarrassment if they are found out, heartache if their love is unrequited. Are they willing to risk it all by opening their hearts and trusting one another enough to fall in love?

I had so much fun writing Dex and Lena's story and I hope you enjoy their journey to their happily-ever-after.

Best wishes,

*Allie*

# A NURSE, A SURGEON, A CHRISTMAS ENGAGEMENT

---

## ALLIE KINCHELOE

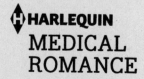

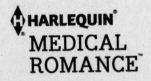

# HARLEQUIN®
## MEDICAL
## ROMANCE™

Recycling programs
for this product may
not exist in your area.

ISBN-13: 978-1-335-14984-8

A Nurse, a Surgeon, a Christmas Engagement

Harlequin Enterprises ULC
22 Adelaide St. West, 40th Floor
Toronto, Ontario M5H 4E3, Canada
www.Harlequin.com

Printed in U.S.A.

**Allie Kincheloe** has been writing stories as long as she can remember, and somehow, they always become romances. Always a Kentucky girl at heart, she now lives in Tennessee with her husband, children and a growing menagerie of pets. Visit her on Twitter: @alliekauthor.

## Books by Allie Kincheloe

### Harlequin Medical Romance

*Heart Surgeon's Second Chance*

Visit the Author Profile page at Harlequin.com.

To all the brave doctors, nurses and other
medical personnel who risk it all each day.

You've inspired me.

# CHAPTER ONE

SCALPEL IN HAND, Dr. Dexter Henry made his initial cut through the abdomen of his patient. As the skin parted, the ringtone he reserved for his mother began to play. His muscles tightened with dread, but before he could open his mouth to tell the nurse handling messages to ignore that one, she read it.

Out loud.

Where everyone in the operating room could hear.

"Dr. Henry, your mother is texting. It says: The Wicked Witch of Westfield will be riding her broom back into town for your brother's wedding. Thought you should know ahead of time. How would you like me to reply?"

Hand frozen over the fresh incision, Dex struggled to maintain focus. The synapses in his brain blasted off like a Fourth of July fireworks display. Jessie had finally resurfaced. For some time now, Dex had managed to put the woman who'd quite literally left him standing at the altar out of his mind. Hearing that she'd returned opened a Pandora's box of memories he'd rather not relive.

Heart beating faster, negative thoughts flashed by one by one like an old film strip in his mind showing him the low points in his relationship with Jessie. It took more effort than he wanted to admit to shove down the moment of panic temporarily overwhelming him. Surgeons with a patient's life in their hands could not afford to let their minds drift off in the middle of a procedure to times—and women—best left forgotten.

"Dr. Henry?" the nurse questioned.

"No reply yet. I'll take care of it when I'm finished here." Dex sighed. Why couldn't his mother have waited until he was out of surgery to text that information?

"Well, now I'm even more curious," the nurse said as she laid his phone back down. "Is there more to you than we know, Dr. Henry?"

Ignoring her question, Dex said, "Suction, please. I need better visualization."

While Dex was trying to put the text and the woman in question out of his mind, the overly eager young resident couldn't seem to let the matter drop. Practically a prodigy when it came to medicine and surgery, the young man had no people skills, and his bedside manner needed work. With his lack of ability to read people squarely on display, the resident pushed for more information despite how Dex had clearly tried to shut the topic down. "Oh, come on, Dr. Henry, you can't leave us hanging like that! Who is the Wicked Witch? Where is Westfield? And most intriguingly, why is it important that you know she's coming to the wedding?"

As the words left the resident's lips, everyone in the room seemed to nod in unison. A chorus of "Mmm-hmm" and "That's right" followed.

Dex closed his eyes briefly. While snapping at the doctor in training might make him feel better temporarily, it certainly wouldn't help this uncomfortable situation. Finally, he decided to give them a very clipped version of his past while keeping his tone ice-cold to discourage further discussion. Still, his secrets would be on the lips of every nurse and carried through the entire hospital on excited whispers by the end of the day. Gossip traveled through a hospital faster than a virus, and he'd rather it be the truth than let them draw their own conclusions from his mother's words.

"Her real name is Jessie. And it's important because she hasn't been back to our hometown since she disappeared on our wedding day."

Only the blips on the monitors and the occasional rustle of paper broke the silence in the OR. The familiar noises seeped into his soul, and he let them soothe the ragged edges that voicing his secrets had exposed. The quiet should have been unnerving, considering everyone in the OR was currently contemplating his confession, but instead he found it comforting. When the silence continued, Dex put his head down and got back to work.

"You know, if you need a date, all you have to do is ask," Belinda finally spoke up.

Who else would make such an offer? Her support brought a smile to his face. Fifteen years his senior, Belinda had taken him under her wing when he'd first arrived at Metro Memorial Hospital with the cocky greenness of residency still permeating his every interaction. She'd taken him down a notch or two. There was no one else at the hospital who he respected more.

"Ah, but, Belinda, I'm already in love with you. Taking you back home to Westfield would just tempt me for things I know I can't have." He winked at the older woman. He didn't

worry that his favorite scrub nurse would mis-
understand his flirty words as an actual come-
on. They didn't have that kind of relationship,
just a teasing dynamic that allowed them both
to let their guards down with each other.

Belinda stared at him over her mask. "If
she's coming, then you need a date."

"It's you or no one, B." Even as the words
slipped past his lips, the truth in her words
sank in. He did need someone to go home with
him for the wedding. Not Belinda, but someone to get his mother off his back. From the
moment his brother Tommy had announced to
the world that Jill had accepted his proposal,
their mother had been on a one-woman mission to find Dex a new love.

His grip tightened around the scalpel in his
hand. He'd rather stab himself with it than give
Westfield something else to gossip about. He
had only been home once since his ill-fated
trip to the altar, and it had been awkward to
say the least. In a single week at home, his
mom had stuck every single woman in town
under the age of forty in his path in hopes that
he'd finally move on from Jessie. Awkward?
Nah… What could be awkward about a parade
of women he wasn't remotely interested in?

He had, though.

Moved on, that is. Even if his mother was having trouble believing that.

He dated. Quite frequently, even. But no one seriously enough to bring home. He only dated to have a little adult companionship on occasion. A physical release, not an emotional connection. No risk for either party. In fact, he told anyone he dated from day one just what he was willing to give, and he always made sure to end things before anyone got hurt. None of the women he'd dated recently would work for this half-hatched plan, either.

He wouldn't want to lead someone on, after all. Taking someone home for a family wedding during the holidays implied so many emotions that Dex almost shuddered in revulsion at the thought. Asking a woman to be his date to a family wedding at Christmas implied that a box with a diamond ring sat under the tree. And he'd never take that step again.

No, he planned to stay single forever. He had zero interest in long-term commitment, and he'd hesitate to do anything that might give any impression otherwise. After his trip down Matrimony Lane had dead-ended with him standing at the altar alone, his entire hometown watching as he got dumped from afar,

Dex could live the rest of his life without putting himself into that sort of situation again.

"Taking a date would save me from more than a few matchmaking attempts and a fair bit of pointed stares. But finding someone on such short notice would be nearly impossible. It's a Christmas wedding," he added aloud, his thoughts running with how much more difficult the timing made things.

Getting someone to pretend to be his new girlfriend in June would have been easy. He'd just spring for a few days at a luxury beach resort and voilà, instant girlfriend. But with the wedding planned for the holidays, it made it ten times trickier to find someone to go along with a fake relationship scheme.

"Ah…so you need someone to go home with you, pretend to like you, and for the holidays no less. That will be hard to find." Lena's green eyes sparkled and he thought he might be able to see a hint of a smile behind her mask. "Who would have thought that a handsome young surgeon would have to resort to a fake Christmas girlfriend?"

"Are you volunteering?" He eyed Lena. She would be perfect. Just his type—long brown hair, more than a few curves and enough sass to keep him on his toes. And even more, Lena intrigued him.

He'd actually asked her out when she'd first started working at the hospital a few months back and she'd turned him down cold. Women didn't tend to ignore him or say no to him. If anything, they usually came to him, leaving him to be the one to let them down easy. But not Lena. She'd looked him up and down, shook her head and said, "I'd rather empty bedpans." Ever since that day, she'd dodged him outside a surgical suite whenever she could.

When she didn't immediately answer, Dex returned his gaze to his patient. "Can I get more suction?"

For the next while, Dex gave his patient and the surgery his full attention. He ensured the patient was taken care of before he returned his attention to Lena.

Making eye contact with her, he murmured, "You never answered me."

Word around the hospital called Lena an ice queen—a brilliant and reliable nurse, but cold and limited in her friendship. He didn't know her story, had no clue why she had icicles in her eyes, but she'd certainly frozen him out. In his eyes, that made her a perfect candidate for a fake girlfriend. She'd never want or expect a proposal under the mistletoe.

Lena tilted her head and stared at him for a moment, her eyes seeming to reach deep into his soul as she considered his question. Scrutinizing him for some time, she finally asked, "How close to Christmas is it?"

"Christmas Eve." He rolled his eyes. "My future sister-in-law is a nut for Christmas. I think she'd have gone with Christmas Day if the pastor at the church would have allowed it."

The smallest laugh came from Lena at his words. "Is she really that bad?"

"You have no idea." Jill lived and breathed Christmas year-round. It had come as no surprise to anyone in the family when the wedding date had been declared as Christmas Eve. No one had blinked an eye since it had been expected from the moment she'd said yes to his brother's proposal. "When you meet her, you'll see."

"When I meet her... When?" She raised an eyebrow and he had to actively force himself not to flinch under the intensity of her gaze. "You're awfully sure of yourself, aren't you? I haven't agreed to anything yet."

"Wishful thinking?" He flashed her a hopeful smile. "It would really help me out."

"Are you willing to return the favor? I have a...thing in Los Angeles on New Year's Eve that would go much more smoothly for me if I had a successful surgeon at my side."

"Are we talking New Year's Eve party or decapitating the one who wronged you?"

Hearty peals of laughter rang out at his dark joke, and an awareness shot up in him like he'd been injected. He shook it off and focused on her words.

"The former. I might have to take you up on the latter, though. It's a fundraiser gala, black tie, of course. My father runs a hospital out there, and lately my mother spends her time doing his bidding and raising money for various charities. If I tell them I'm coming alone, it will be, uh, very strongly suggested that I take my father's current protégé as my date. And if there's anything I want less than attending this gala in the first place, it's attending it with *that* guy."

"Well, I do happen to own a tux. I suppose we should coordinate the details sometime before then." The dark-haired surgeon glanced over at her, and she thought he might be smiling beneath his mask. "It wouldn't be good if my fake Christmas girlfriend missed the wedding because I didn't give her the right directions."

Thank god for surgical masks that hid the blushes that her body seemed determined to produce any time he glanced her way. What was wrong with her? The man made her crazy. She couldn't be in the same room with him without wanting to strangle him, so why did she find herself glancing in his direction every few minutes and growing warm whenever their eyes met?

"So, who here is skipping the hospital Christmas party on Saturday?" the anesthesiologist asked. "I'm on call so I'll have to be here even though I hate the Secret Santa crap. Who needs another Christmas candle or a gift card in a lesser denomination than you brought? Or worse, a polo shirt that's three sizes too large, like I got last year."

"I'm skipping it," Lena and Dex said at the same time.

"Ooh… You two have a hot date?"

"No." Again, they spoke at the same time. Dex looked over at her and their gazes locked over the patient. A hint of amusement crinkled the laugh lines at the corners of his eyes.

When she met his eyes, though, her heart grew erratic. Dr. Dexter Henry had eyes a woman could spend the rest of her life lost in, with thick, dark lashes that framed them perfectly. But more than being captivating, those eyes held a level of emotion Lena wasn't used to seeing. A hint of mirth sparkled over his little joke, but behind that lingered a shadow. Had the ex-fiancée put the darkness in his gaze? And what would it take to banish the ghosts of his past and brighten his eyes back to their true brilliance?

"Uh-huh." The anesthesiologist laughed. "It would be more convincing if the pair of you weren't sneaking heated glances at each other every few seconds and practically finishing each other's sentences."

Lena shook her head, unable to form words at that moment. If other people were noticing, she must have been looking at Dex far more than she'd realized. Embarrassed tears welled up in her eyes and she blinked rapidly, determined to keep them from spilling over. *Crap.*

Gossip had been the motivating force behind her leaving LA, and she'd been in Nashville less than six months before finding herself right back in the middle of it. The one-year contract was supposed to give her the breathing room she needed to decide what to do with her life. Nashville had started to feel like home.

Despite its lack of sand and ocean views, she could see herself making a life there. Away from California and her overbearing parents. She'd found a calm in Tennessee, but the anxiety and fears that the fresh start had quelled came rolling back in with a vengeance when she found herself the topic of conversation again. She swallowed hard. She hoped no one noticed the big, shaky breath she took while trying to gain control over her emotions.

"Leave it alone, Jason," Dex warned, his voice low and firm. "Worry about our patient, not my personal life."

"Come on, Dex, I'm just having a little fun. Don't get your scrubs in a knot."

"It's not fun for me, and I don't think it's fun for Lena. So knock it off."

An inexplicable urge to hug him rose up, and she had to squash it before she made an even bigger fool of herself. Past experience had taught her that men got close to her for one reason—to get close to her father for his connections in the medical field. She had never had a guy stand up for her just for her own sake, and it gave her this warm, fuzzy feeling deep down inside.

She tried to avoid looking at him and only spoke when necessary while they finished up the gallbladder removal. The puzzle of how Dex benefited from standing up for her rolled around in her mind unsolved.

The more she'd thought about it, the more she worried there was too much at risk. And she was the one who stood to be hurt. She'd been told how he'd dated half the nursing staff. A doctor could do that, though, whereas a nurse could not. She needed to put a stop to this before they reached a point of no return.

After surgery, she found herself alone in the scrub room with Dex. They washed up next to each other without speaking. She dried her hands and stepped away.

Lena took a deep breath and glanced at the door. She should really make her escape before she got sucked deeper into this ill-fated charade and the man at the center of it. Something about Dex had drawn her like a moth to a flame when she'd moved to Nashville. Handsome, of course, charismatic even, but something more about the young surgeon called to her. A confidence in his gaze that pulled her in like gravity and made spending time with him a risky endeavor.

After one surgery with him where she'd had to stand tucked at his side, arms brushing as they moved for several hours, she'd known they'd be physically compatible if nothing else, so when he'd asked her out, she'd shut him down hard. Getting involved with him was a risk that she just was not willing to take.

She'd heard the rumors about him. According to hospital gossip, Dr. Dexter Henry got around. His motto seemed to be love them good and leave them quick. His type was *exactly* why she'd uprooted her career and moved across the freaking country, after all. She'd fallen for the playboy once and still had the scars on her soul as souvenirs. Swallowing hard, she pushed those thoughts to the far recesses of her mind.

Lena couldn't take the risk of real involvement. Not after the things she'd seen when a relationship went wrong. So despite the surface-level attraction she felt to Dex, she'd never let it become more. Ever. After the fallout that had followed when the truth about her relationship with Connor had surfaced, Lena's entire foundation had been shaken. Her career had nearly collapsed back in California. The negativity had invaded all aspects of her life and convinced Lena to stay single for the rest of her life. Unfortunately, her parents were not on board with Lena's plan for an eternity of lone wolf status.

Statement of fact—she needed a good-looking, successful doctor to go home with her. Bringing home a date who looked like Dex might be the only chance she had of getting her parents off her back when it came to dating Martin. They'd been pushing that angle since about ten minutes after the scandal about Connor broke, and she'd love to avoid it if she could. Her dad had deemed his protégé to be perfect son-in-law material, while Lena herself would rather gnaw her own arm off than to marry, or even date, that balding schmuck with his fake tan. Her mother wanted her to settle down with Martin because it would force Lena to return to LA because of his career.

Dex presented a nearly perfect solution to the Martin situation. With just one problem...

"I'm not sure how nosy your family will be, and maybe with the wedding taking some of the focus off, we can get by with your family easily, but my family will expect me to know you if we are dating. Really know you. I don't bring a lot of guys home, so—"

"What do I need to know?" Dex interrupted her to ask.

Visions of Dex being the guy to make Martin disappear and get her parents off her back vanished with the delivery of that single question. As the only daughter of William Franklin, an egotistical plastic surgeon turned hospital administrator who thought himself better than every female in his acquaintance, Lena had spent much of her life being treated like her voice was nonexistent. Connor had been the same, but she'd been so stupidly in love with him that she'd overlooked his every fault. It wasn't until they'd broken up that she'd decided she'd never voluntarily spend time with a man who didn't have enough respect for her to allow her to finish speaking again, and she didn't plan to change her mind now. Even if Dex was the most likely candidate for helping her to avoid her parents' attempts at marrying her off.

"First of all, I absolutely cannot stand being interrupted like that. So if you aren't going to let me speak or if you are going to insist on talking over me, then we should both find someone else." Lena's eyes narrowed as she glared at him. With her fists balled at her sides, she added through clenched teeth, "You will be respectful enough of me to wait until I have finished my sentence or you can try your best to find another woman willing to pretend to be your girlfriend for this wedding, are we clear?"

Satisfaction rushed over her when Dex gaped at her for a moment. "Yeah, I'm sorry."

Lena's head moved side to side dismissively. "Why do guys do that? Do you even *realize* that you do that?"

"I'll try to be more mindful."

Tiny little wrinkles appeared on his forehead as he seemed to sink down into his thoughts. They made Lena wonder if anyone had ever pointed out to him that he talked over them. Or maybe she had merely projected some of her frustrations onto him. Either way, she kind of liked seeing that she'd gotten his attention. It had made him think at least a little about how he treated women. She'd never managed to accomplish that with her father or Connor.

"Okay, so as I was saying," she continued. "I don't bring a lot of guys home. My parents will assume that we are fairly serious if I have brought you home for the gala. Because of that, they will expect that you know things about me, things a dating couple would know. More than we can cram into a couple of plane rides. The best I'll be able to tell my family is that you are right-handed but prefer to keep your tools on the left for some unknown reason and that your favorite sandwich seems to be the turkey club since you've had it three times a week since we met. We need to spend some time together and learn these things."

"Are you asking me on a date, Lena?" The confusion on his face had cleared. In its place sat a self-satisfied smirk.

*And there it was.*

That unbearable arrogance that all the surgeons she'd ever met possessed. Her father had it in spades. Connor had thought far too much of himself too.

Was it issued to them along with their medical license?

"Ugh!" Her hands flew up in irritation. "Why did I ever entertain this idea?"

Annoyance flashed through her, white-hot and simmering on the cusp of anger. Dexter Henry made her crazier than anyone had in a long time.

"Because you know we'd be perfectly suited to take care of each other's needs." Not a question. There was an undercurrent to his words that took that phrase from simple statement to sensual promise. His gaze moved over her body before he made eye contact once more, making her one thousand percent certain that he'd meant his words to have multiple meanings.

Her skin heated under the scrutiny of his gaze and she swallowed hard.

She couldn't do this.

No way. She could not spend two weeks with an arrogant man who changed women more than a lot of nurses changed their scrubs, but worst of all, made her want him to take off his scrubs and see if he could live up to the masculine sexuality he projected. Even if he won in every category when compared to Martin—better hair, nicer smile, sexier... Nope, she wasn't going continue that line of thought. Shaking her head, Lena took a step back.

"This is a bad idea."

*Or a very good one...*

"Hear me out before you reject the idea entirely."

She waited for him to speak, crossing her arms over her chest. He'd need a good pitch to get her sold on this idea. He was far too much temptation for her otherwise.

"We both need a significant other to get us through the holidays unscathed by the cupid wannabes in our families, right?" He raised an eyebrow and waited for her to nod before he explained, "As far as I can see, neither of us has another solid lead on that."

"Having you with me would help me avoid yet another matchmaking attempt." She sighed.

"Like I said, though, my family will expect us to know things that dating couples would know."

Not having to be partnered with Martin for another fundraiser would save her feet a great deal of pain, though. Her parents had insisted that she attend a gala with him at the local children's museum. The clumsy plastic surgeon not only had two left feet, but a complete inability to recognize his lack of skills. He'd nearly crippled her before she'd thought of a plausible excuse to leave early. But dancing with Dex would be dangerous for other reasons. She wasn't sure she could keep her distance from him if she had to step into his arms. And getting close meant risk. Her goal was to get through the New Year's Eve gala with as little risk as possible.

"So, we tell them that we only met a few months ago, which is the honest truth, but then tell them we started dating fairly recently but things are getting serious fast. That will help us with the not knowing enough details about each other. No one will expect us to know everything there is to know after only a couple months of dating."

"I don't know." She chewed on her lower lip.

Dex's plan made a lot of sense, but she worried about spending so much time with him.

"Come on," Dex coaxed, his voice lowering as he tried to sway her decision. "What do you say? You go to the wedding with me, I'll go to the gala with you, and then we conveniently break up a few weeks into the new year. No one in either family is the wiser for it."

"Okay," she found herself saying. She almost couldn't believe she would be taking a man home to meet her parents that she'd barely had a conversation with. Remembering how her dad had grilled Connor the first time she'd brought him home, Lena shuddered. "There may be a pop quiz, though."

Not that her father's interrogation had sidetracked Connor's plans… He sold himself to her father with the same charisma he'd used to charm her. Lena had fallen for him quickly and her parents had been just as taken. It was only once Connor had gotten what he'd wanted— her father's influence to gain a promotion— that his true colors began to show.

"Luckily, I'm a good test taker." Dex winked at her, causing her stupid heart to somersault inside her chest.

*Dex Henry is not datable.* She repeated

the little mantra to herself. *Dex Henry is not datable.*

"This isn't a joke." Lena put her hands on her hips and frowned at him. She tried to focus on the frustration she felt for Dex, not the attraction, but the hint of a smile that played on his lips distracted her more than she wanted to admit even to herself. "I don't know why I'm agreeing to this if you aren't going to take this seriously."

"I'm very serious, Lena. You know what? I think I'm going to have them leave you on my service through Christmas. It will keep us together during the days and give us some legitimate things to talk about. The fewer lies we have to keep straight, the better, right?"

"True." He certainly had a point on keeping things as close to the truth as possible.

"How about some dinner? We can discuss the finer points of our agreement." He raised a brow in question.

She shook her head. "No, if we are doing this, we are keeping it quiet around here. I do not want to be counted as the next notch on your well-whittled bedpost."

"Okay then. I've got patients to check on."

He looked a little hurt by the brusqueness in her words, but recovered quickly. He stepped past her without another word.

# CHAPTER TWO

"GOOD AFTERNOON, MR. CLEMONS." Lena moved into a patient's room, pushing a medication cart. "Looks like you should get to go home later today, according to your notes. I've got your afternoon meds, and if everything goes okay for the next couple hours, you are out of here."

The old man in the hospital bed perked up at her voice. "Ah, but my beautiful Lena, when I go home, I won't have anything so lovely to look at as your smiling face."

"Flattery will get you everywhere. You want an extra Jell-O? Some ice cream? I'm your girl." She smiled at the patient as she scanned his wrist band for the medications. "Now, here are your meds. I have a painkiller and an antibiotic."

His age-spotted hand shook as he took the tiny cup. "Ice cream does sound good."

"Take your meds first and I'll get you some

in just a few." She watched as he tossed the pills into his mouth and chased them with some water from a Styrofoam cup. She made a note that he had taken the medications. "Chocolate or vanilla?"

"I've always been partial to chocolate. Are you married, my love?"

"I'm not, never found a man like you." She patted his arm. His chart said he was single. "What about you? Ever married?"

"No, I never did. I came close once, probably quite a few years before you were born, but…" He trailed off. He shook his head and a wistful look came into his eyes. "Eh, you don't want to hear this old man's tales of woe and despair."

Lena pulled up a chair. "If you want to tell me, I do."

She'd learned years ago that sometimes the most important thing a nurse could do for a patient was to listen to them. Even if it didn't seem relevant to their current condition, or medically related at all, the act of engaging in a meaningful conversation created a bond, a trust, that encouraged the patient to be honest. And that was most certainly relevant.

"It was a long time ago. Her name was Betty. She had blond hair and the prettiest smile I've ever seen—I'm sorry, my love, but even prettier than yours—and after our first date I knew that she was the only woman I'd ever give my heart to. After our third date, I bought an engagement ring. That was two weeks to the day after we met."

Lena laughed. "Whirlwind romance, huh? Do you really think you can know that fast if something is meant to be?"

He took her hand in his. "My dear, if you don't know by then, you aren't with the right person."

Lena let that statement sink in. She'd never felt that before. Even with Connor, who she'd been in love with. And she thought they'd moved fast; after all, it had only been a month after they'd started dating that he'd been pushing to meet her parents and talking about forever…

A forever that was never meant to be.

"So, what happened with Betty?"

He sighed. "That third date was a double date with my best bud and his girl. I dropped Betty off at home and went and bought a ring. Even woke the jeweler up so I could get it—there weren't any twenty-four-hour-type places back in those days. I called her the next morning to try to set up another date, and her mother tells me that Betty had run off to get married."

Lena's jaw dropped. "What?"

He looked out the window, the slightest hint of tears shining in his eyes. "Seems she liked the look of my buddy more than she did me. They eloped. Married forty-eight years when she died last year."

"Oh, Mr. Clemons, I'm so sorry." The bulge in her throat was hard to choke down. This was why she didn't date anymore. Why she didn't trust. Even when someone was supposed to love you, so many times they were just waiting for a chance to hurt you. She'd learned that lesson the hard way.

"I never met another who made me feel half of what I felt with her."

What would it be like to trust someone enough to feel twice what she'd felt for Connor? It was unfathomable to her. Connor had thrown her life into such turmoil. And the lack of familial support in the matter had caused her to shut down even further. If you couldn't even trust your own parents, well, what was the point in sticking around? Hearing her dad side with Connor after the breakup had been the final straw.

After months of dating, months of hearing her father praise Connor and not so subtly put her down in the same sentence, Lena really should not have been surprised when her father continued to treat Connor like his future son-in-law, despite all that he'd put her through. When she'd told her parents that things were over with Connor, neither offered her any condolences. Instead, she was questioned on what she'd done wrong to lose him. After all, a surgeon like Connor was a stretch for a mere nurse like herself. So it must have been her fault.

If there was one thing Lena knew, it was how to be alone. Even if some of her "alone" had been when in the midst of her family. Her heart hurt for the sweet old man sitting here. No wife, no children. He hadn't even had a visitor that she'd seen. "So you've been alone all this time?"

"I've lived a long life. I had a long and accomplished career. I've just outlived everyone in my life." He patted her hand. "Don't be sad for me. I'm not sad for myself."

She couldn't help but be sad for him, though, and sad for herself. Even if they'd both made the choice to live their lives without anyone else involved, loneliness wasn't an easy cross to bear. Tears pricked her eyes and she blinked furiously, determined not to cry in front of a patient.

"I'll be right back. I promised you a chocolate ice cream, didn't I?"

Before leaving the hospital for the evening, Dex wanted to check on his patients. He had residents whose job it was to follow up after surgery, but he liked doing it. Many of his patients he barely saw before taking them into the OR. He whistled a low tune as he walked up the hallway toward his first patient's room.

Lena was coming from the other end of the hall, talking to another nurse. He was really baffled by her. Normally, women liked him. But not her.

She challenged him. And he liked it.

An alarm sounded at the nurses' station and Lena and the other nurse ran toward one of the rooms.

Over the PA system came a call for help. "I need a crash cart and the code team to Three North. Code team to Three North. Code Blue."

Dex wasn't on the code team, but he moved to the room in question. He grabbed gloves and pulled them on. "How can I help?"

Lena and the other nurse were moving around the patient. Lena pulled the pillows from beneath his head and lowered the bed to a flat position. The heart monitor showed a very weak, irregular pulse—V-fib—and the blood pressure monitor beeped to alert to the patient's low pressure.

Not one of his patients, Dex was relieved to see.

The other nurse began chest compressions. "Can you intubate him?"

Lena pulled out an intubation kit and handed it to him. She laid an Ambu bag out next to the man's side.

The patient's eyes were closed, his skin already showing the graying of lack of oxygen. The only movement to the man's body was from the compressions of the nurse.

Dex moved quickly, inserting the tube in the man's throat so that they could breathe for him. As soon as he removed his hands from the tube, Lena connected the Ambu bag and started squeezing it, forcing air into the man's oxygen-deprived lungs.

Still the monitors remained chaotic. The heart rate did not change. In fact, it seemed weaker. CPR continued.

The code team rushed into the room, slamming the cart into the wall in their rush. The doctor running the code took over. "I'm Dr. Clark. I'm leading this code. How long's he been like this?"

"About two minutes, Dr. Clark. Should we give him epi?" Lena asked.

Dex couldn't help but admire her professionalism in the chaos of the room. While people were darting quickly here and there, Lena was a calmness in the eye of the storm. She alone seemed unflappable in the moment.

"Yes. One milligram of epi." Clark reached for the paddles. "Charge the defibrillator. We are going to have to shock him and see if we can get his heart back into rhythm."

A moment later, the beep indicating the defibrillator was ready sounded. "Okay, everyone clear. Shocking."

The heart monitor went from jagged spikes to a total flat line.

"Asystole," Clark said, even though everyone in the room could read the monitor. "Push another round of epi."

He charged the defibrillator once more. "Okay, everyone clear."

The man's body jerked from the power of the shock. Still, the monitor showed only a flat line. No peaks, no valleys. This man wasn't coming back. And to keep trying would only be a waste of time and resources.

Clark hung the paddles back on the crash cart. He checked for corneal reflex. Tried for a pulse. And last took his stethoscope and listened for breath sounds. Shaking his head, he said, "He's gone. Time of death: six twenty-one."

Clark and his team left the room as quickly as they had entered. And in the space of a breath, the chaos from before was gone.

Lena switched off the machines one by one. The room fell into silence. There was a calm that seemed odd when contrasted with the flurry of noise and movement just moments before.

The other nurse laid a hand on Lena's shoulder. "I'll make the calls."

Lena shook her head. "There's no one to call. No family, no friends. He was all alone."

"Funeral home then." The other nurse shrugged and left the room.

Lena took the Ambu bag and tossed it. She removed the tube from the man's throat that Dex had placed. She started cleaning up the paper wrappings and remnants of trash left from the code. She pulled the electrode pads from the man's skin and put them in the trash too.

Dex wasn't sure she realized he was still in the room. She looked utterly heartbroken. The strong, unshakable nurse he'd been admiring during the code had been replaced. Now the woman in front of him looked like she might burst into tears at any given moment.

"Mr. Clemons, this wasn't how today was meant to end. You were supposed to be going home." She sniffled. She smoothed the old man's hair back. "I thought we were going to have ice cream together. I even brought your favorite—chocolate."

"Are you okay?" he asked.

She jumped at the sound of his voice. "I thought you'd left with the others."

"I wanted to be sure you were okay first."

"Of course I'm okay." The paleness in her face disagreed with her words, though. "We lose patients all the time. He's not my first, and I know that unfortunately he won't be my last."

"You look shaken by this one, though," Dex argued.

"If I'm ever not shaken when I lose a patient, that's the day I quit, because I will have lost more than my patient." She started disconnecting all the monitors and IVs attached to the now deceased patient.

"Shift's almost over. Have dinner with me?" She looked so upset about losing this patient that he didn't think she should be alone tonight. He'd always thought of her as this ice queen, too cold to feel, but seeing her like this made him wonder if maybe his preconceived notions about Lena were entirely wrong.

Lena looked like she might argue, but then she nodded. "Okay. Dinner sounds good."

"I'll meet you out front in twenty?"

# CHAPTER THREE

AT A FEW minutes after seven, Dex rolled to a stop in front of the main entrance of Metro Memorial to wait for Lena. He bumped the heat up so that it would still be warm inside the car after she'd opened the door. The mid-December day had been crisp and cold. The freezing chill and icy wind that cut straight through a person made him glad he'd sprung for the upgraded package when he'd bought the SUV. Those heated seats were worth every extra penny.

Lena came out the door wearing only scrubs, rubbing her hands briskly up and down her bare arms. Puffs of her breath rose in front of her in the frigid evening air.

*What is she doing out in these temperatures without so much as a sweater?*

He pulled up right in front of her. Lowering the window slightly, he called over the wind whipping around the buildings and cars,

"Hey, Lena, I'm here. Come on, get in out of the cold."

Hurrying over, Lena climbed inside. "Hi," she said, her teeth chattering as she shivered.

"Where's your jacket?" He reached over and turned her heated seat on. "It's freezing today. You're going to get hypothermia."

"I, uh, don't have one yet."

He stared at her, unable to speak for a moment while he tried to process her statement. Her eyes were puffy like she'd been crying. He wanted to ask if she was okay, but he didn't want to overstep. So he decided to focus on the immediate concern she'd presented him with.

"It's December. What do you mean you don't have a jacket?"

"It's my first winter here. I wasn't sure what the climate would be like. And I didn't know it was going to go from shorts weather last week to snow flurries almost overnight. Isn't Tennessee supposed to have four seasons?"

Dex snorted. "Yeah, it does. Winter, pollen, suffocating heat and fall."

"I missed fall."

"It was only three days this year. You might have worked through it."

"Winter wardrobe is on the list for my next day off." She shrugged as she put her seat belt on. "I never understood why so many cars had heated seats, but now I'm thinking they should be standard equipment."

"You came from LA, right? Is that where you grew up?"

"Oh, yes. My father runs a hospital now, but he spent years as the most sought-after plastic surgeon for the stars. My mother spends all her time working charity events and fundraising." Melancholy tinged her soft sigh. "My first boyfriend was a celebrity's son, and we broke up when he asked me why I didn't ask my dad to 'do my tits' for my birthday because he found mine a little disappointing."

Hearing the indignation and more than a little hurt in her voice, Dex glanced over to Lena. She had her arms crossed across her middle, unintentionally pushing her chest up. He grunted. "He's an idiot. I see nothing that would disappoint me. I hope you told him that he should see your dad for a bit of enlargement action of his own because he was the disappointment."

She chuckled. "There may have been comments along that line. It was our last date."

"Jessie was my first girlfriend." The confession tumbled past his lips.

"The ex-fiancée?"

"Yeah. That's the one."

"How long were you together?"

"Almost nine years." And now they'd been apart almost as long.

"Wow."

Pity permeated that single syllable. The same pity he'd heard in every single condolence after Jessie had disappeared. It had pervaded the looks in people's eyes and filled conversations that stopped when he walked into the room. His hand clenched around the steering wheel.

Swallowing hard, he gave Lena more details than his brief admission in the OR had provided. "I found out she left the state while I was standing in the church, greeting the guests we had invited to our wedding."

"She left you at the altar? That's harsh."

"Yeah." He hadn't been in love with Jessie for a long time now. But man, that punch to his pride was hard to get past. "After our rehearsal dinner, I kissed her goodbye. She got into her mother's car and drove away. Sometime during the night, she disappeared."

The cracks in their relationship had shown before that fateful night, though. Dex had just been too stubborn to see it. Jessie had struggled with the hours he'd put in during med school and had for some reason convinced herself that he'd be done as soon as he graduated from medical school. They'd fought over his hours a lot—she accused him of being a workaholic, when really he'd passed up surgeries and procedures in an effort to spend more time with her and avoid even more fights. She'd never understood his need to be a doctor, but seemed to like the idea of being a doctor's wife. He'd thought they'd be okay once he got through his residency. They didn't make it that far.

"Did she ever tell you why she changed her mind?"

He shook his head. They'd shared a lot of dreams that Jessie had walked away from without a backward glance. The swift way she'd cut all ties to him told him all he'd needed to know about their relationship, or lack thereof, really. After all, a person in love didn't ghost the person they were in love with, so clearly Jessie hadn't been in love.

"Nope. I have some assumptions, of course, but we actually haven't spoken since that day."

"I can't imagine spending nearly a decade with someone and walking away like that."

Dex puffed out a breath. "She doesn't seem

to have looked back. But that's the past. Can we please discuss something besides how my first love ripped my heart out and tap-danced on it in front of literally every single person that mattered to me?"

Lena seemed to shrink back a bit from the vehemence that leaked into his voice. "So, where is Westville?" she finally asked.

"Westfield," he corrected, far more gently than he'd spoken to her before. "I'm sorry if I'm snappy about Jessie. Every time I go home, my mom starts trying to pair me up and bore witness to me being left at the altar. That wound is still a little raw."

"The breakup or the embarrassment over it?"

He didn't have to think about that answer. "The embarrassment, for sure. Jessie and I would have never lasted, even if we had gotten married that day. The pain of the breakup itself is long gone. I'm not pining for her, if that's what you are wondering, but the embarrassment just never seems to fade."

"Gotcha," she said softly. "So, taking me home with you is about more than blocking a matchmaking attempt. It's about showing all your old friends and neighbors that you found someone new."

"Yeah," he agreed. That was exactly it. Every time he spoke to someone from Westfield outside his family, inevitably they brought up the fact that he'd been left at the altar. It had become a never-ending horror story. "So, Westfield is a few hours' drive east of here, a small town nestled in the Smoky Mountains. Population about eight hundred."

"Wow." Lena snorted. "My graduating class had over nine hundred people. I'm not sure I've ever even been to a town that small."

"City girl," he said with a teasing tone.

"You have a little accent when you say *girl*," she said, poking his arm playfully. "Did you realize?"

A laugh rumbled up from deep in his chest. "Honey, if you think I have an accent now, wait 'til I'm around my family for a few days. All the *y'all*s and dropped letters will seep back in and I'll sound like the biggest hick you've ever laid eyes on."

"Don't call me honey."

"If you don't like being called honey, you moved to the wrong state." He pulled into a parking space in front of a steak house that wouldn't raise an eyebrow at Lena's scrubs. "Is steak okay? We can go somewhere else if you prefer."

"Steak's good."

He turned the ignition off and hopped out. The concrete walkway glistened with thousands of little ice crystals. Before he'd made it to the front of the SUV, she came up next to him, shivering. He slipped his blazer off and draped in over her shoulders.

"When we get to Westfield, I'm going to need you to sit in the car and wait for me to open your door. My mama raised me to be a gentleman and I'll catch hell if you don't let me treat you like a lady. Now, watch your step on this sidewalk, it's a little icy."

She raised an eyebrow at him and pulled the blazer closer. "You gave me your jacket. Isn't that gentlemanly enough?"

Stepping forward to open the restaurant door for her, Dex laughed. "Only someone not raised in the South could say something so naive. According to my mama, a man can never be gentlemanly enough."

Lena stepped through the door, her eyes twinkling with amusement. "I don't know if I'm the right fit for you to be bringing home to *mama*, then."

He told the host they needed a table for two before turning back to his conversation with Lena. "Why the negative emphasis on 'mama'?"

"I've never heard a grown man call his mother 'mama' in conversation like you just did. Most people of my acquaintance would say 'my mother' or 'my mom.' And I know no one who is grown and still says 'mama.'"

"Men of your acquaintance. Do you know how prissy that sounds?" He waited while she slid into the booth and then sat across from her. "It's a Southern thing, I guess. If I call her 'Mother,' she's going to tell me to stop sassing her and maybe box my ears for me."

Lena held the menu up, her eyes scanning down the list. "If I called mine anything but 'Mother' she'd give me a lecture about how my informal attitude could create negative impressions of our family. And nothing upsets Vivienne Franklin more than negative impressions." She slammed the menu down on the tabletop. "Unless it's my father creating that negativity. And then she will ignore it as if it never happened."

"Guessing there's a history there?"

"My father—" The server came over and Lena cut off her answer midsentence.

After they'd placed their order and were once again alone, Dex prompted her, trying to get her to tell him what she'd meant about her dad. Her actions said there was a story there, one that would be important for him to know.

Anger flashed in her eyes when she looked up at him and confirmed his suspicions. "I don't want to talk about it."

Frustration welled up within him at her words. They were here because she said they needed to get to know each other. And now she didn't feel like talking?

"Hmm…" Dex leaned back against the padded back of the booth and stretched his legs out, trying hard to project a calmness he certainly didn't feel at that moment. "So, what do you want to talk about? Getting to know each other better was *your* idea, after all."

"I know. And I'll tell you about my father before we go to LA, I promise, but for now, can we just start with something lighter? That conversation will simply make me angry, and I don't want to be angry tonight."

"One last question and I'll leave it alone." He waited until she nodded. "Why do you feel so obligated to go back for this gala? Seems like it would be less stress to just skip it."

"Family obligations. Now, can I please change the subject? Today has been—" she paused and seemed to roll a few words around before deciding on the right one "—hard. So, we should probably set some guidelines about this, right?"

"Probably. My brother's wedding is Christmas Eve. It's been strongly suggested to me that I arrive at least a couple days before and stay through the holiday. How's that work for you?"

"I'm off from December 19 through January 6. I had the dates put into my contract because I knew I'd never get the holidays off otherwise, and my mother will make life unbearable for me if I don't attend the gala."

"And the gala is on New Year's Eve?"

She nodded. "I think we can both agree that we need to keep the PDA as minimal as we can, stick as close to the truth as feasible, and once we get back from LA this is done. And I think the fewer people at Metro Memorial who know about it, the better. Neither of us needs anyone to think that we are hooking up."

"Simple enough," he agreed. "Should we shake on it?"

Wrinkling her nose, she ignored his outstretched hand. "I don't feel that's necessary. Less physical contact is probably the best course of action, don't you think?"

"Okay, then." He didn't quite agree, but he

let her have this one. "And I think no emotional attachment is a pretty obvious one. Anything else?"

When she shook her head, he brought the conversation back to getting to know each other by asking, "So, what brought you to Nashville?"

Lena grumbled low enough Dex didn't catch her words.

"What was that?"

Her fingers traced little designs in the condensation on her water glass, and he thought maybe she was going to blow off another answer, when she finally did speak. "A relationship gone horribly wrong and my freaking father's inability to be faithful to my mother— both of which ruined not only my personal life but spilled over into my professional life as well."

"That sounds like a loaded topic."

Her bottom lip quivered a bit and she sucked in a shaky breath. But thankfully, she didn't burst into tears. He wasn't so great with tears.

"He makes me so angry I can barely think straight."

"Your dad or your ex?"

"Both." She shrugged. "My ex only dated me because I was the medical director's daughter and being with me got him closer to the man who could—and did—advance his career."

"How long ago did that end?" The wound still seemed raw from his perspective. He just wasn't sure which man had caused her the most pain.

"April."

Less than a year. Considering the timeline, Lena was doing far better than he'd been at the same point. Jessie had broken him for a long while. He could relate to a relationship gone wrong if she'd just open up and tell him about it.

"And your dad?"

"My father, well, other than repeatedly cheating on my mother with women half his age—including my best friend while I was dealing with the worst breakup of my life, by the way? He's a cold, overbearing jerk who expects total obedience and has standards so high that an Olympic high jumper couldn't reach them."

Clearly any conversation about her family would be a touchy one. He couldn't quite decide if she was more angry or hurt by father, but their relationship wasn't good. What sort of dad slept with his daughter's best friend?

And for that matter, what sort of friend slept with their best friend's dad? Was the friend climbing the career ladder by climbing Lena's father? He'd ask, but Lena had made it crystal clear that she was ready for happier topics.

He'd struck out on trying to start a conversation twice. Maybe the third time would be the charm and he'd finally get some insight into what made her tick.

"Are you an only child?"

She nodded. "I am. What about you? I know you have a brother since you need a date for his wedding. Is it just the two of you?"

Her answer was exactly what he'd expected to hear. The familial obligation he'd only seen with only children. People with siblings, in his experience, were more likely to tell their parents when they needed to back off and would even walk away if it became necessary.

"Oldest of three boys, actually. The one closest in age to me, Tommy, is getting married to the literal girl next door. And I should probably go ahead and tell you that Jill is my ex's younger sister."

Lena raised a brow in surprise.

"Small town." He shrugged.

"Does that bother you?"

Tommy had asked him the same thing before he'd ever asked Jill out the first time. He couldn't blame Jill for Jessie's actions, though. That wouldn't have been fair to her. "Nah. Jill is nothing like Jessie. And if my brother is happy, then I'm happy."

"You said there were three of you?"

"My baby brother, Wade, is a senior at the University of Tennessee this year."

"I always wanted a brother or a sister." Wistfulness softened her voice. "But apparently I did so much damage to my mother's figure that she was unwilling to do that again."

Dex desperately wanted to lighten the mood. He tried a little joke. "You can have one of mine. I have a spare."

She snorted at his offer, and he could see she was trying desperately to hold back a smile.

The laughter in her eyes contradicted everything he thought he knew, and she was quickly becoming a code he was determined to break. Behind the laughter, there was a sadness that lingered in her eyes, and she often looked like she held the weight of the world in her slim fingers.

He wanted to make her smile for a bit. To chase the shadows out of her gaze and hear her laugh while she relaxed in his arms.

* * *

Lena shifted and her leg bumped into Dex's under the table. Even sitting in a booth, he had managed to spread himself out and take up so much space. The way his shoulders filled out those navy-blue scrub tops had fueled more than a few fantasies since she'd moved to Nashville. She fought against a blush as the memory of one of those fantasies popped into her mind.

Even in scrubs, Dex oozed masculinity. Tonight, in khakis and a button-down shirt, an air of power surrounded him, not unlike what she'd come to associate with her father and her ex-boyfriend. But with Dex, she didn't feel like being female made her less.

She'd have to examine that thought in more detail when Dex didn't sit so near she could barely breathe. She'd been hoping to find something about him that she hated. Some little detail that confirmed her suspicions of him being too much like her father, maybe. Or anything that reminded her of Connor allowing her to push him firmly back onto the "men she'd never date" list.

Dex was in line to be head of general surgery when the current head retired. It was common knowledge at Metro Memorial that Dr. Miller had been grooming Dex to take his place by letting Dex take a leadership role within the department. Like her ex, Dex would be in a position of power. In a decade, he'd be running a hospital, just like her father. Powerful men caused powerful problems for the women in their lives. Lena could not allow herself to forget that.

But here he sat, smiling that gorgeous smile of his, doing something incredibly sweet by offering to share his siblings with her. While he surely meant it in a teasing way, she couldn't help but find the gesture endearing.

What was wrong with her?

"It's so kind of you to share," Lena deadpanned.

Dex laughed. "Consider it self-care. If he has someone else to pick on, then I get a break."

The delicious sound rolled over her, tempting her to want things that a fake relationship could never provide. Lena swallowed hard, fighting to regain her control and perspective. Fake meant she walked away unscathed. Real meant the consequences were equally as real. And she refused to do real.

"Which brother are you talking about?" She needed to get the conversation on something light, something that wouldn't be too tempting, because she couldn't take much more tonight. If he pushed her one way or the other, she might break.

"Both." He shrugged. "Either. You'll see when we get to Westfield."

"Tell me about them. Or about your parents," she suggested. Dex didn't seem to mind talking about his family. Starting there meant she didn't have to open up just yet. She'd left LA to get away from the embarrassment of everything that happened with Connor and her father and to escape his influence, and bringing them up and talking about their actions felt like tempting fate and potentially destroying even more of the peace she'd found here in Tennessee.

While they ate, Dex launched into a lively description of his parents and his hometown, and Lena had to squash down the envy. His narrative portrayed the idyllic childhood she'd only seen on television. From hiking in the Smoky Mountains with his parents, to trying all the touristy attractions in the area, every story spoke of a family with a solid and loving commitment to each other.

By comparison, her family had been a dysfunctional mess hidden behind a cosmetic front of perfection. Their family vacation spots were chosen for their exclusivity and her parents' enjoyment, never her own. Memories of her parents involving her in any sort of family-style entertainment slipped through her mind like wispy clouds pushed by a stiff breeze. When none cemented into a solid recollection, she released a deep sigh.

"You don't have a single bad story, do you?"

Dex had the type of family Lena had always wanted. When Dex talked about his family, love warmed his voice like a perfect cup of hot cocoa, and Lena had never had that. Might never have that if she couldn't find it in her to trust a man enough to have a family.

"Uh... Nothing much. We've had our squabbles through the years, but what family doesn't? Nothing we couldn't work out." He grinned at her. "There was this one time that my dad and I..."

Dex launched into a story about how he and his dad had pulled a series of pranks on his younger brothers, and her heart hurt. She'd be willing to bet that his father would never have slept with a woman under his employ, nor ruined the woman's career when the relationship went sideways. And from his description of his mother, she'd bet Mrs. Henry would not have ignored being cheated on and certainly would never have just gone on with her life as if it never happened. The man sitting across from her would never have to fear what his own father might do to his career, and he'd certainly never have to move across the country to get away from his father's influence.

But the worst part, the part Lena was really struggling to reconcile, was her dad sleeping with her best friend. During the absolute worst months of her life, she'd had no one to talk to. Her mother turned her away, dismissing her and her emotions like an unwanted telemarketer. And her best friend, the girl she'd grown up with and trusted with all her secrets, had slept with her father until he tossed her aside like yesterday's leftovers. And so then Lena had lost her best friend as well. It had been a long and lonely spring for her and she'd jumped into the travel nurse gig without a second thought—anything to get her away from California and the negativity that abounded there. Her memories weighed heavy on her, her heart aching like she'd been stabbed.

Swallowing hard, she blinked hard at the tears that all the thoughts of her upbringing and more recent turmoil had brought up. As she blinked, a tear dripped from her eye and slid down her cheek.

She should have canceled this fake date. Her nerves were already on edge after losing Mr. Clemons this afternoon, and her emotions couldn't handle being this close to a man like Dex—completely her opposite in so many ways and yet somehow drawing her in like waves to the shore.

Despite a smooth surgery with Dex, her day had been a roller coaster full of unexpected twists and emotions. A sweet elderly man had come through surgery yesterday looking like a champ, only to code that afternoon on her watch. He'd been alone, never married, no children, and it had hit Lena hard that she was staring down her own future. The thought hit her again that she might never have a child of her own, and her lower lip quivered.

"Hey, are you okay?" A warm hand covered hers.

Embarrassment washed over her. She met his gaze, feeling super self-conscious about how he caught her mired in the depths of her thoughts. "Yeah, sorry. I got lost in my own head for a minute."

Worry highlighted the gold flecks in his dark eyes. The weight of his hand over hers was warm and solid. Comforting. And when he spoke, his soft tone soothed her more than the teasing words themselves could have ever done. "I've never bored a woman to tears before."

"Well, you can't say that any longer." She laughed as she swiped at the stray tear on her cheek.

"Wanna talk about what's really bothering you?"

She searched his face, surprised to find genuine concern there. "Not at the moment," she finally answered. "Your childhood sounds perfect."

"I was lucky." His thumb rubbed circles on the back of her hand until she pulled away. That simple touch sparked a far too tempting awareness that radiated from the skin on her hand all the way down deep into her core. The attentiveness he showed was quite honestly the most irresistible feature she'd seen in a man in a long time now.

She needed a distraction. Something to take her mind off how every nerve in her body stood up and took notice of his touch. A television mounted to the wall behind him played a professional basketball game. She focused her gaze on the screen while she tried to pull herself together. Usually she could stare at something from a distance and put her emotions in check in the process. But this time, it wasn't working. Not even a little.

"I'm sorry. Could you take me back to my car?" She covered her plate with her napkin. She had to get out of there before she lost all control over her emotions. "I'd really like to go home."

Shock briefly crossed over his face before he schooled his expression back to neutral, but to his credit, Dex didn't question her decision to end their evening. He merely waved the server over and asked for the check. Within a couple minutes, they were out the door and on the way back to the hospital.

Several times, she saw him glance in her direction as he drove. He had to be thinking she was a nutjob. But she was on the verge of tears and she did *not* want to break down in front of him. And if she didn't get away from him soon, that's exactly what would happen.

"Where are you parked?" he asked as he turned his SUV into the parking garage.

"Exit side of level three."

When they got to her level, she pointed out her car and he slowed to a stop near her trunk.

"Thanks for dinner," she murmured, reaching out to grab the door handle.

"Hang on a second." Dex hit the lock button to keep her door from opening.

"What are you…?" She stared over at him in confusion.

"I thought tonight was going well, but then you just shut me out." His frustrated sigh filled the SUV. "What happened back there? Did I do something wrong? Say something that upset you?"

Lena shook her head, trying hard not to cry.

"I'm trying to wrap my head around how this went downhill so fast. This isn't going to work if you don't talk to me. We go see either of our families like this and it's gonna look like we've been fighting the whole trip."

"I know. I just…" She choked back a sob. If she started crying, she might not be able to stop. Holding it together until she got away from him was the only hope she had to keep from embarrassing herself beyond recovery. "I can't tonight, Dex."

"Okay, well, if you aren't in, if you can't stand to be around me for even a single evening, then let me know, sooner rather than later, because I need time to come up with a new plan before Tommy and Jill's wedding." When she nodded, he unlocked the doors. "Good night, Lena."

She moved to shrug out of his blazer and he stilled her with a hand on her shoulder.

"Keep it until you get your own. You need it more than I do right now."

She got out of the SUV and closed the door. Dex waited until she'd gotten in and started her car before he pulled away.

Sitting in her car, she sucked in several deep breaths. She tried to be strong, really, she did, but now that she was alone there was no stopping the tears. They burst out of her like water spilling from a dam, cascading down her face. She leaned her head against the steering wheel and let the sobs punch through the remnants of the walls she'd surrounded herself with.

Today had taught her something—she did not want to spend the rest of her life alone, even if she had argued that point with her parents more than once. She didn't want to be eighty and have no one to miss her when she was gone.

A rap on the glass sent her heart straight out of her chest and into orbit.

She trembled as she looked toward the window at her side.

*Dex.*

He yanked the door open the second she hit Unlock, grabbing her hand and tugging her out of the car and into a gentle embrace. "Tell me what I did to cause this. Lena, I really have no idea."

She swiped at her tears with the sleeve of his jacket. Great, not only was Dex witnessing her breakdown firsthand, he thought he'd caused it.

"That patient we lost today," she found herself confessing on a sob. "It was like looking at the Ghost of Christmas Future—no family, no friends, just him alone and dying at Christmas with no one to miss him when he was gone."

"That's not your future." Dex pulled her in closer. She sank into his warmth, her heart fluttering at his nearness. His touch made the world around them fade, and suddenly the future seemed less bleak. He murmured reassurances as he rubbed his hand up and down her back. "One day you will find someone who makes your heart skip a beat. He'll sweep you off your feet when you least expect it. You won't be alone. I know it."

Why did he have to be such a nice guy? Making it through the next two weeks at his side would be a lot less scary if he wasn't the antithesis of everything she'd assumed he'd be. Yes, he was arrogant and powerful. But he was also thoughtful and kind. He came back after dropping her off to make sure she was okay and if that wasn't a sign of true character, she didn't know what would be.

As a result, a single question currently dominated her mind—if Dex treated a virtual stranger like this, how would he treat the woman he gave his heart?

## CHAPTER FOUR

A FEW DAYS LATER, Dex wandered around Green Hills Mall, looking for the perfect Christmas gifts for his family. He normally made sure to get his shopping done long before Thanksgiving and the nightmare of Black Friday, but time had gotten away from him this year and with less than two weeks before Christmas, he'd had no choice but to make another attempt at the mall in December. The memory of the little old lady who had not only snatched a sweater out of his hand but then smacked him with her purse for protesting held a spot in his mind any time he got near a crowded mall, even though years had passed since that incident.

Just stepping through those automatic doors sent his pulse pounding in his temples. His breathing grew shallow and rapid and he had to wipe his now sweaty palms on his pants leg. He could walk into a complicated surgery without an ounce of nerves, but a busy shopping mall sent him into an uproar.

Dex swallowed hard as a woman carrying multiple bags while talking very loudly on her cell phone walked right into him and shouted at him to watch where he was going. He bit back the retort that jumped to his lips because she moved on without a backward glance.

Why hadn't he just ordered everything online and had it delivered? He shook his head and kept moving. The thought that it wasn't yet too late to do that sprang up in his mind, at least not if he was willing to pay through the nose for expedited shipping.

"Dex?"

He spun when he heard his name called, but when he saw no one that he recognized, he returned his attention to navigating the crowd surrounding him. Only a few gifts, then he could go home.

"Dex!"

Once again he heard his name and stopped to look around.

"Dex! Look up!"

From the upper level, he saw a familiar face staring down at him. "Wait right there," she called. "I'll come to you."

"Lena!" He moved around a group of grandmothers toward the escalators, and he and Lena met next to some potted plants just out of the flow of foot traffic. "This place is a madhouse. Why would anyone come here?"

The smile on her face could have lit Westfield for a month with its brightness. "Oh, don't tell me you are a Scrooge!"

He narrowed his eyes at her. Beaming with happiness, Lena looked perfectly relaxed and much happier than the last time he'd seen her. The brightly patterned scarf draped around her neck would have looked tacky on him, but on her it was perfection. Christmas spirit vibrated off her palpably.

His future sister-in-law would love her.

"You are already watching all of the Christmas romance movies and listening to Christmas music all the time, aren't you?"

She motioned him closer.

When he bent down a bit at her coaxing, she tiptoed and mock-whispered in his ear. "It's the most wonderful time of year." Her lips brushed his ear on the last word and a shudder of desire sliced through him as sharp as a scalpel.

"Is it?" He rested his hand on her waist, his head still bent near hers. Tension sizzled white-hot between them and had him wondering if they could turn this time-limited charade into a time-limited fling. The physical novelty always wore off quickly for him and he lost interest in the women he'd dated after a few weeks. It would surely be the same with Lena, but they could still help each other out in the meantime.

Lena remained on her tiptoes. Their faces were millimeters apart. But just as he pulled her closer, someone jostled into them and Lena moved away. Her cheeks flushed bright pink.

"Um…" she began, but then trailed off.

The moment might have slipped away, but Dex didn't want to let her slip away. "Would you like to help me with my Christmas shopping? I'm sure you'll be much better at it than I am, and your presence will make this day far more bearable."

People moved past them, many chatting with a friend, some alone moving faster as if on a mission. Christmas music played loudly through speakers overhead. Dex only had eyes for the beautiful nurse standing within arm's reach, wearing his blazer with the sleeves rolled up.

Biting her lower lip, Lena looked at him as she seemed to consider his offer. "What if we run into someone from the hospital? I thought we were going to keep this on the down low?"

"So, I tell them I am a hopeless shopper and bribed you into helping me." He sweetened the offer. "Lunch is on me. We can discuss the next two weeks and work out any kinks."

"Deal." She stuck her hand out to shake.

As their palms met, Dex had to suppress the urge to pull her back into his arms. After how fast she'd shot away from him, he didn't think she'd be eager to fall right into his embrace. And he didn't want to scare her off after they'd seemed to make a tentative truce the other night. Something had changed after her emotional purge, and she'd started to open up to him the tiniest bit more, at least when she didn't realize she was doing so.

And if he frightened her away, then he'd have to go home alone for his brother's wedding. He'd never find anyone else this close to Christmas to pretend to be his girlfriend. According to his dad, there would likely be a repeat of the eligible ladies' parade if his mom had her way. And he certainly didn't want to have to face Jessie alone. That would be so awkward.

Not that he was still hung up on his ex.

At all.

Jessie had killed any and every feeling he had for her when she'd walked away without a word, leaving her father to come to the church and break his heart. To his dying day, he'd never forget the look on Ray's face when he'd told him Jessie had left town. "I'm sorry, Dexter, but her note only said that she wasn't ready to get married."

But he knew how it would look to the people of Westfield if he showed up alone. They would assume he still pined for her after all this time. They would assume that he had hopes of a Christmas reconciliation.

Nothing could be further from the truth.

In reality, he just hadn't found anyone he was willing to risk his heart on again. Getting left at the altar could really do a number on a guy—even if he had been the tiniest bit relieved once the shock wore off. He realized just what a bullet he'd dodged in being left at the altar; it was far better than marrying someone who really didn't want to be married and going through a bitter divorce later.

But falling in love with a woman gave her a power over a man that Dex wasn't sure he could ever give again. It wasn't that he didn't believe in love or anything as harsh as that. He just didn't believe that love was ever in his plans again. Short-term flings with no feelings involved kept him satisfied and his heart protected.

"So, what are we looking for?" Lena questioned, pulling his thoughts away from Jessie and the past. "I'm just looking for some winter clothes. As you reminded me, I'm not exactly equipped for a Tennessee winter." She plucked at the lapels of his blazer, her radiant smile giving him stirrings of thoughts toward the future. "And I thank you for the loan again. It came in handy in the just above freezing temperatures this morning."

"I bet it did," he said with an easy smile. "I think I might like how it looks better on you than me anyways."

The tiniest hint of pink brightened her cheeks again but she met his gaze. "I don't know if I'd agree with that, but it's certainly warm." She held up the bags in her hands. "I found some warm sweaters, but I haven't been able to find a winter coat yet that I like."

"Maybe you are just too picky?" he teased, loving the reactions he coaxed from her with a few words.

She wrinkled up her nose. "Maybe I just have more refined taste."

He took the bags from her hands and nodded in the direction of the nearest store. "Well, we won't find you a coat without looking. Have you been in there?"

"That was actually going to be my next stop."

She allowed him to guide her into the store, where she made a beeline for some ugly Christmas sweaters. Picking up a green one that was nearly the color of her eyes, she held it up in front of her. "We should get these for your brother's wedding! What do you think? Is this one me?"

"I think Jill would kill us. At least for wearing them to the wedding. But I might buy her one of these for a Christmas present. She'll love it."

Lena laughed, but stopped suddenly. She tilted her head, and her expression grew thoughtful. "You know, I never asked how fancy the wedding was going to be. Do I need something formal?"

Dex shrugged. "I have no idea. I was told to bring my black suit. And Jill has, apparently, picked out matching ties for us all."

"Yeah, men have it easy. A black suit is appropriate for anything casual to dressy. It's not so easy for us girls."

It couldn't be that hard. Dresses were the female equivalent of a suit, weren't they?

"Just wear a dress."

"Dresses come in various degrees of formality and to wear the wrong one would be a massive faux pas." The expression on her face said he might have been the one to make a massive faux pas. "What did the invitation say?"

"I didn't get an invitation."

She gaped at him. "Why are you attending a wedding you weren't invited to?"

"I'm not allowed to say no, so there was no need to waste money on an invitation for me."

"Then how am I supposed to know what would be appropriate for me to wear? I don't want to wear something casual and find out everyone else is formal, or even worse, wear something more formal than the bride herself." She shuddered in apparent horror.

"I could call my mama and ask her," he offered, trying to figure out what he needed to do to fix this before the entire situation derailed.

His offer seemed to be the right decision because Lena perked up as he spoke. "Have you told them you were bringing a date?"

"Not yet. I wanted to be sure that you were coming." He rubbed the back of his neck. Suppressing a shudder of his own, he let his mind wander to his family's reactions if she didn't go after he'd told his family she would be there.

His brothers would never let him live down getting stood up again at a wedding, even if it wasn't his this time. His dad would just shake his head and possibly give him a talk about what to look for in a "good" woman. And his mom? She'd worry herself into a frenzy about him being alone for the rest of his life before launching herself into a mission to have him married off by May. "The only thing worse than showing up alone would be to say that I was bringing someone home with me and *still* show up alone."

"True."

"Have you told your family that I'm coming?" he asked, turning her question back around on her.

With a sigh, she shook her head. "No. Like you said, I wanted to make sure it was going to happen first."

"Well, I'm committed to you."

The words came out without thought and he almost apologized for the bluntness he'd put on the statement. It had sounded rather like an accusation instead of the motivational comment it should have been.

The din surrounding them almost drowned out her reply when she said softly, "I'm committed too."

* * *

Lena slipped into the fitting room to try on a few items of clothing while Dex called his mother to check on what exactly she should wear to the wedding. Through the slats on the door, she overheard every word of his conversation. His deep voice carried even over the Christmas music piped in from above.

"Hey, Mama," he said. "Yeah, I miss you too. I had a reason for calling actually."

He either paused or moved away.

Lena stopped moving with a pair of gray corduroy pants halfway up her thighs, listening carefully as she tried to catch Dex's next words. Eavesdropping unashamedly, she stood half-dressed in the fitting room without moving a muscle so that she could better hear Dex over the sounds of the store.

"No, I'm not calling to cancel just because Jessie is coming. I was actually calling to make sure it was okay if I brought my girlfriend with me."

The smile that sprang up on her lips at the word *girlfriend* surprised her. She yanked the pants up and looked at her reflection in the mirror. When she realized why she was grinning like a fool, the smile quickly became a frown. Being called Dex's girlfriend shouldn't make her smile.

It was fake. Their entire relationship was fake.

She shoved the pants off and roughly hung them back on the hanger. She didn't even try the pair of khakis on and just put her own jeans back on. Her desire to shop had fled with the realization that she'd really liked hearing Dex refer to her as his girlfriend. She had to get her head straight and remember that, even if Dex wasn't quite as bad as she thought, getting involved for real would ruin everything that she'd accomplished by leaving California.

She knew this with every fiber of her being.

So why was she having such a hard time remembering that when Dex was around?

Putting on the coat she'd picked out, she examined her reflection. It would do for now. She didn't have the luxury of waiting for the perfect piece of outerwear to come along.

Once she had dressed, she stepped out of the fitting room and almost walked right into Dex. He seemed to be pacing back and forth in front of the fitting rooms. Agitation deepened the frown lines marring the perfection of his face. A muscle twitched at the corner of his eye and a rigid grimace darkened his countenance.

"Mama, I told you, it has nothing to do with Jessie. I want you guys to meet Lena and—" He stopped suddenly like his speech had been interrupted on the other end of the line. After a lengthy pause he answered, "Yes, ma'am. No. She's right here if you want to talk to her."

Before Lena could squeak out a protest, Dex had shoved his cell phone into her hand. "I can't do it anymore. You talk to her," he grumbled before stomping away, his shoulders squared off in visible frustration.

"Hello, uh, Mrs. Henry," she said, hoping she wasn't about to get cussed out by some crazy Southern woman she'd never met. Getting told off before they'd even met just might be the icing on the cake of this charade they'd made inescapable when they involved his mother. She didn't expect his mom to love her, or anything of the sort, but if his mom hated her, it would make for a long and stressful week in Westfield.

"My son tells me you are coming home with him for Christmas and Tommy's wedding."

The voice on the other end of the line was as stereotypically Southern as any that Lena had ever heard faked out in LA.

"Um, yes, ma'am, I am. If that's okay with you, that's the plan."

*Suck up.*

She was totally and completely sucking up to his mother. What was wrong with her?

"Do you work at the hospital with Dexter? I know that son of mine and if you didn't meet at the hospital, then you'd have had to trip him at the grocery store to catch his attention."

Lena couldn't help but laugh. "Yes, we met at the hospital. I'm a registered nurse."

"I see. You don't sound like you are from around here."

"No, I'm from California."

Mrs. Henry snorted. "Well, I suppose I won't hold that against you. If Dexter's bringing you home, he must see something special in you. He hasn't dated anyone in years that was serious enough for him to bring home to meet the family."

"I… Um… I don't think I'm that special."

She knew the truth. Dex wasn't bringing her home because he thought she was special. He was bringing her home because he needed a pretend girlfriend and she fit the bill. The hope she heard in his mom's voice hurt. They were going to get her hopes up that Dex was seriously in love with someone, and for what?

"Oh, well, Dexter thinks you are, and I trust my son. I'm so excited to meet you. Dexter has been alone far too long and it does my heart good to hear that he's found someone to love. Maybe we will have more than one thing to celebrate this Christmas!"

His mom seemed so genuinely warm and kind. And completely enamored with the idea of Dex settling down with a new love. A huge lump of guilt rose in her throat and Lena had to choke it down. Deceiving his family left a bad taste in her mouth, but she'd made a commitment to Dex to be his pretend girlfriend through the holidays and if she was anything, it was stubborn. She'd see this through or die trying.

Forging on out of sheer determination to keep her word, Lena continued the charade but changed the topic to something less likely to trigger more guilt. "I had asked Dex what I should wear and he sputtered something incoherent that I took to mean he had no clue. A few suggestions would be appreciated, if you don't mind?"

A short chuckle met her ear. "That boy wouldn't know a tea-length dress from a ball gown. The wedding isn't going to be very formal, though. They are going with a rustic holiday theme, complete with burlap lace. Anything dressy you feel pretty in that doesn't show off all the goodies God gave you would be appropriate. And the rehearsal dinner is going to be an ugly Christmas sweater party. So if you want to bring something hideous for that, my soon-to-be daughter-in-law will find that illogically delightful."

Another smile crept up on Lena's face at the revulsion she heard in regards to the ugly sweaters. She thought the gaudy Christmas sweaters were fun, but Dex's mother clearly did not agree. She nearly snorted when she pictured her own mother's face if anyone dared wear one of the Christmas sweaters to one of her charity events—it would be epic.

"Sounds great. I'm sure I'll find something appropriate for both the wedding and the rehearsal. Thank you for the tips. I look forward to meeting you soon."

"And the same to you, dear. Tell my son to call me later, would ya?"

"Of course."

Lena hit End on the call and looked around for Dex. He had stopped pacing and slumped down onto a bench outside the fitting rooms.

"Here's your phone back." She held it out for him to take as she stepped over to him. "Your mother wants you to call her later."

"Did she say why?"

"Well, she seemed to think I must be something special if you were willing to bring me home. Her exact words were, 'Maybe we will have more than one thing to celebrate this Christmas,' if that gives you some idea where she's taking this."

He threw his head back into the wall so hard Lena heard the thump. "She didn't," he said with a groan.

"Oh, yeah." Lena sat next to him and nudged his side with her elbow. "And she's so excited that you're in love again."

Dex huffed out a noise of disbelief. "I can't believe she said that."

Lena leaned against him, her shoulder pressed against his biceps. She looked at him out of the corner of her eye and couldn't resist a bit of a tease, hoping to get a rise out of him and distract him. "If you don't freak out and confess our plans, I think we really can pull this off."

"I hope so." Dex didn't take the bait. Instead, he took her hand in his and Lena squeezed his in solidarity.

"We got this." Trying a different tactic, she infused her voice with positivity. "We will go to Westfield and they will think we are so in love that we will be announcing our own wedding once it won't steal your brother's thunder."

With his thumb rubbing slow circles against the back of her hand, Dex exhaled long and deep. "And when the truth comes out, they will never forgive me, will they? What are we doing? Is salvaging a little pride for one day each worth potentially hurting both of our families?"

Worry and concern roughened his voice and gave her a minute's pause.

"Listen, we've already told your mom that I'm coming. If I don't show up now, I think that will make things worse for you, won't it?"

Dex murmured something noncommittal that could have been either an agreement or a disagreement.

"If they don't know our relationship is fake, it can't hurt them, right? Seriously, we just mention each other for a few weeks after the holidays and then casually say we broke up. No one gets hurt. That's what you told me, remember?"

Why did it feel like she was the one talking him into this mess now?

"Right." They made eye contact and a lingering spark in his gaze smoldered brighter as they continued to look at each other. Smack in the middle of a crowded shopping mall, with "Rudolph the Red-Nosed Reindeer" playing through the overhead speakers, a spark fluttered between them. The place buzzed with Christmas spirit, frazzled nerves and people going further into debt, but Lena's eyes seemed locked with the handsome surgeon's next to her.

"So, remember those sweaters we saw on the way in? We are totally buying those for the rehearsal dinner." Lena stood and held out her hand. "Come on. I'm starving and we have gifts to buy."

# CHAPTER FIVE

THE WAY HER cheeks pinked up when he pulled out her chair made him want to do more for her. Something about that shade of pink made him think about what he could do in order to see it again. *And if that isn't crazy...*

Once they got through the holidays and this fake romance, Dex needed to find someone new. Someone who didn't want forever and who didn't look at him like he was a jerk for only wanting short-term. He hadn't had a deep connection since Jessie. In fact, he'd actively avoided making a connection that lasted longer than a month. But why did that seem less and less appealing?

"So, why did you become a doctor?" Lena asked as he rounded the table and sat across from her.

"I wanted to help people."

It wasn't the greatest of answers, but it was

an honest one. Maybe a little bit of an over-simplification, but true, nonetheless.

She snorted. "Nice try, Doc. I'm gonna need a bit more info than that."

"Long story short, when I was ten, I witnessed a really bad car crash. And the paramedics, they were just brilliant. I watched them take these people that were so bloody, I thought they had no chance. And they pulled them out of this mangled heap of metal and got them in an ambulance."

She tilted her head and stared, eyes full of questions. "So why not a paramedic?"

"Honestly, that's what I wanted at first. I even did a couple ride-alongs, but it was a paramedic that convinced me to go to med school. He told me that surgeons were the ones who really helped the most people. So I got involved with this mentor program that let me shadow a couple surgeons for a day, and, well, the rest is history."

That conversation that day in the back of that ambulance had been life-altering for him. It had set him on a trajectory out of the tiny town of Westfield and into a life that he loved. Westfield had been a great place to grow up, but he'd had little problem leaving it behind.

She wrinkled her nose in disagreement.

"Clearly that man has never worked with a nurse. Because all nurses know who really helps the most people as well as keep the hospitals running."

Dex laughed, both at the cockiness in her voice and the truth in her statement. Years ago, he'd learned that if a doctor got on the wrong side of the nursing staff it made for a rough work environment. Nurses definitely made the world go 'round and kept a doctor's arrogance firmly in check.

Still, he couldn't just admit that to her, could he?

"Yes, we know, nurses are the real rock stars. Yet how many nurses can perform something as simple as an appendectomy or save a person from a ruptured spleen?"

Lena rolled her eyes. "Point taken. We are all necessary."

"Anyways, so then I set my sights on being a surgeon. And that's my story." He paused and looked around the crowded restaurant. Red-and-gold tinsel hung from the rafters. Why did every place insist on burying their business under a rainbow of Christmas trappings?

When Lena didn't continue the conversation, he did. "Why did you become a nurse?"

"Because it angered my father." She snatched

one of the rolls from the basket the waiter was setting down. "At least initially."

They quickly ordered, and Dex tried to steer the conversation back to her motivations for being a nurse. He straightened in his chair and leaned forward with interest to catch her answer. He'd known a lot of people who took jobs for various reasons, but to spite their parent? That was a new one.

"You chose a career simply to tick off your dad?" He held back the laugh that tickled against his lips because the expression on Lena's face was one hundred percent serious. Deep in his gut, he knew laughing now would be one of the worst mistakes he could make with the beautiful nurse sitting across from him.

She picked bits off the roll, smooshing the tiny bits of bread between her fingers. "My father is one of those doctors who thinks nurses are second-class citizens. You don't do it, but I know you've seen the kind I mean. That act like nurses are only there to do their bidding."

He nodded, pulling in a slow breath and releasing it even slower while he thought of the best way to respond. Lena was the definition of someone with daddy issues, that much was clear. She'd need to let go of all that if she wanted to truly move forward.

Lena continued without his response, though. "In my misguided youth, I thought that if I were to become a nurse, I could show my father that nurses were worthy of respect."

He let the statement settle and it felt heavy. The weight she carried around with that mission meant she was far stronger than he'd given her credit for. Every scrap of information he learned about her ticked his admiration up a notch or two.

"And how'd that work out?"

She laughed sadly. "Not well. But it was absolutely the best decision I've ever made. I love my job."

"You're really good at it too."

Her cheeks pinked up again but she met his eyes when she said, "Thank you."

Dex took a big gulp of water, swallowing hard. Lena was so much more than he had been expecting. Being around her made him oddly nervous. He worried she'd see his hands shake or realize that he had butterflies constantly flitting about in his stomach when he was with her.

He'd saved lives. Taken organs out of people's bodies. Sliced through layers of skin and muscle. He'd held a human heart in his hand during a cardiac rotation and massaged it back to life. Going on a fake date with a beautiful nurse should be as simple as pie.

Lena's heart raced as Dex complimented her. Knowing your skills and having them recognized by someone else were totally different. She wasn't sure she'd ever stop blushing when someone praised her. This was starting to feel a little like a real date, though, and she felt the need to rein it back in.

The waiter brought their food by and then once again left them alone.

Lena poked at her food for a minute, rolling ideas around in her head for how to begin this conversation. "So, um, we should talk about expectations."

"Seems simple to me. You pretend to be my girl while we are in Westfield for a few days for my brother's wedding. I'll pretend to be your guy while we are in LA for your fund-raiser thing." He jabbed a fry in her direction. "No emotions. No risk. Simple enough."

Lena patiently took a large drink of her water. "I meant the finer points of the agreement. Logistics, travel dates, lodging."

He popped the fry in his mouth and chewed,

his eyes never leaving hers. "I figured I'd sort out the details for my thing, you'd sort them for yours. But I really like your concern for our sleeping arrangements."

The air between them seemed charged with that hint of this being more. His voice wrapped around her and sent zings of electricity up and down her spine. She swallowed hard, trying to put the picture out of her mind of them sharing a bed.

"While I think that's an acceptable start, I'm really going to need more details. I need to know where I'll be staying while we are in Westfield."

"With my parents, of course. My hometown isn't exactly set up for out-of-town visitors. It's more of an idyllic haven in the midst of a tourist area. There are no hotels in town, only some rental cabins. The closest are down the mountain in Gatlinburg."

"With your parents?" She gulped.

"Yeah. But it'll be fine. They have a spare bedroom and I'll be in my own room next door."

The odd feeling the settled in her chest in that moment took Lena some time to identify. It was a mixture of relief and disappointment.

How bizarre that she should feel disappointed about the idea of her own room.

"Unless you'd rather share," he said with a wide grin.

She took a large bite and chewed slowly while digesting that line of thought. The blatant flirting she could deal with, but she didn't like how her body reacted to it. Not giving in to the temptation that Dexter Henry presented was going to be a big challenge.

It was hard to keep her eyes off the handsome surgeon sitting across from her. And when he flirted, it made her think about things she had no business even imagining. Dex could break her heart if she wasn't careful. But she was done being this submissive nothing, catering to the whims of surgeons who thought themselves better than her.

And she wasn't going to give him the chance to hurt her.

Even if they had so much chemistry that she found herself daydreaming about just how much Dexter Henry was her type. Because she didn't have a type anymore. That implied she could trust someone enough to let them in.

And the last thing she was willing to do was to trust another surgeon.

"No, my own room is an inflexible requirement. My parents have several spare rooms, if you want to stay at the estate. I'm happy to foot the bill for a hotel while we are in California, though." She took the emotion out of her tone. This was a business transaction, nothing more.

"You decide. I trust you." He leaned across the table as he said it, taking her hand in his.

Lena's breath shook when she inhaled sharply. "I think we need to keep the PDA to a minimum too."

He held on when she tried to tug her hand away. "We have to be comfortable touching each other, Lena. We'll be in close proximity and under scrutiny. Even if we say minimal touching, there has to be some. Or we will be fast outed as fakes."

Shifting uncomfortably in her seat, Lena still tried to tug her hand free. "Maybe so, but do we have to do this now? I could eat easier if you weren't holding my right hand hostage."

"Fine." He squeezed her hand before letting it go. "But you know I'm right."

"Do you worry about them finding out that this is all fake?" She changed the subject, refusing to discuss the idea of them touching further in that moment. "My family will be critical, examining for weaknesses in our story and cracks in our relationship, in hopes of it not working out so that they can continue to push me toward marrying a man of their choice."

Dex leaned back and shook his head. "Why would you let them tell you who to marry?"

Lena stared down at the melting ice in her glass. "You don't understand the pressure. Sometimes it's easier to give in than to fight and fight only to lose anyways."

"Some things are worth fighting for." He reached out and ran a finger down her arm gently. "Like love. You can't help who you love, Lena. And you sure can't let someone else decide that for you."

"Oh, believe me, love is not a factor in their decisions."

"Well, my mom's just going to be happy that I'm seeing someone. She won't expect perfection."

"I feel a little guilty deceiving everyone." Lena sent him a wry smile. "Don't you?"

He shrugged. "Maybe a little. But it benefits both of us, and if we do this right, it's not like they will even know. No one needs to know, and that way no one gets hurt."

She nodded an agreement, but couldn't help but think that the person most likely to get hurt in all this was her. Sucking in a deep breath, she focused on the positives.

"We did manage to get a lot of shopping done today. How about a wrapping party to get all these gifts ready for our trip?"

"Whatever makes you happy," Dex said, staring her down.

Lena licked her lips under his scrutiny. She could think of a lot of things that might make her happy right now, and every single one of them involved a certain dark-haired general surgeon.

She was in so much trouble.

# CHAPTER SIX

DEX RECLINED BACK on the couch, feeling the tension ease from his muscles. He flipped on the hockey game and tossed his phone onto the table out of reach. He was half-asleep when a loud banging came from the door.

It sounded like someone was kicking it?

He answered the door and his jaw dropped. "Uh, how did you know where I live?"

"Belinda told me." Wrapping paper and ribbon filled Lena's arms. From the various angles her rolls projected from her grip, it looked like she had a very precarious hold on the colorful load. She was grinning from ear to ear and her cheeks were as bright a shade as the paper in her hands. "Are you going to let me in or not? I'm about to drop all this all over your doorstep if you don't."

"Yeah, of course." He jolted into movement and pushed the door open wide, motioning for her to come in out of the cold. "Can I help?"

"I think if you try to take any of it, I'll drop it all." She stepped over to his coffee table and squatted down. She carefully dropped all the festive trappings across the wooden surface. A spool of silvery ribbon bounced off the table and rolled across the carpet to his bare foot.

"What is all this?"

She waved a hand vaguely at the mess she'd just made of his coffee table as if that was explanation enough. "We're wrapping presents tonight. I told you this."

"I got it covered." Dex gestured toward the hearth where a stack of gift bags sat beside the presents he'd purchased with Lena's help. He didn't wrap presents. Gift bags were made for a reason, the reason being that wrapping paper was an unnecessary annoyance created to annoy people who weren't overflowing with Christmas spirit.

"I have presents in my car too. I couldn't carry everything at once. Since you don't have shoes on, I'll get them myself."

"Lena…"

But she had disappeared out the door before he could verbalize another thought.

She came back a moment later with several bags in her hands. She set her bags on the couch before turning to him, hands on her hips. "Did you forget that I was coming over tonight?"

"I didn't think you were serious!" Dex protested against the accusatory tone in Lena's question. He'd thought she was joking when she'd said she'd be at his door with bells on to wrap the gifts they'd bought before they left for Westfield in a couple days. He never expected her to actually show up with wrapping paper and ribbons.

"I'm always serious when it comes to Christmas!" Spinning around, Lena's eyes took in the minimalistic decor. A measure of shock shone brightly on her face. "Why don't you have a Christmas tree?"

Dex huffed. "Because I'm a busy surgeon who lives alone and won't even be in town for Christmas? What's the point?"

She looked so affronted by that he decided not to tell her that he'd never once had a Christmas tree in this house. She might implode. At the very least, it would launch her into another rant about Christmas spirit and the importance of the holiday season.

The last tree he'd put up had been with Jessie the Christmas before their disastrous attempt at a wedding. She'd moved from Westfield to live with him in Florida while he finished med school. He'd hoped that by removing the physical distance between them, the emotional one would close too. Their relationship had been splintering even then, but he'd stubbornly tried to patch it like a crumbling gingerbread cookie. The thought of losing her had propelled him into proposing, and her acceptance had been half-hearted at best. He'd been too bullheaded to even allow the idea that Jessie didn't want to marry him into his head. In hindsight, he'd lost her before that Christmas, and all the Christmas traditions and wedding planning had only pushed her farther away.

He'd spent every waking moment of that December planning a wedding with a woman who'd been apathetic about the idea at best. It should have given him pause, but no. He'd prodded and planned while she seemed more interested in watching breakup movies and going out with her new friends without him. Reflecting back, he couldn't remember why he fought so hard to keep their relationship intact when it had been clear she was pulling away. Or why he had let it get so far without addressing it at all.

Instead of communicating concerns, he'd pushed her to get married, somehow thinking a ring would be the glue that held them together. He'd ignored the hard signs of trouble, how her eyes constantly drifted to other men, how she never wanted him to touch her, how she had zero interest in planning their wedding. She'd wanted the world and he'd been working as hard as he could to try and give her those dreams.

Looking back, he could pinpoint his being matched to the residency program in Nashville as the final straw for her. That notification had come in the week before their planned nuptials and she'd actually cried. For the first time in a while, Jessie had shown emotion. She'd wanted him to request a different residency program. Preferably something on a beach, she'd begged, but anything that got them out of Tennessee. The signs had all been there. He'd just been too stubborn to see them.

A poke to the belly brought his focus back to the present and the woman standing in front of him. "Well, where's your tree? We'll put it up."

He rubbed the back of his neck and winced as he said, "I don't have one."

At her gasp of horror, he struggled to hide a smile. Maybe celebrating Christmas again wouldn't be so bad if it meant getting a reaction out of Lena. Her face was so expressive that he wanted to keep pushing her, to see if her eyes sparkled with anger like they did with amusement.

"We will just have to go out and buy you one. Where are your shoes?"

"Tonight we are wrapping presents, right? We won't have time to do that and go get a tree and decorate it. I have to be at the hospital at five in the morning for back-to-back surgeries, so I need to get some sleep at least."

Although she wrinkled her nose, and he could tell she wanted to protest, she finally agreed. "I want it noted, though, that wrapping presents without the presence of a decorated tree might be against the rules of Christmas."

"There are no rules to Christmas."

"Of course there are rules to Christmas." She rolled her eyes. Pulling her phone out of the back pocket of her jeans, she pulled up a music streaming app. When a Christmas carol blared out of the device's tiny speakers, she sat the phone on the table next to the ribbons. "Like, you have to play Christmas music while you decorate. Also when gifts are being wrapped. Preferably with eggnog?"

He shook his head. "No eggnog either."

"You have to have eggnog." She strode into the kitchen and flung the refrigerator open.

The sigh she released as she stood in front of his open refrigerator sounded frustrated. "Not even boiled custard? You really are the Grinch in human form."

"You know the Grinch didn't actually hate Christmas?"

Crossing her arms over her chest, Lena faced him down, clearly ready to hand him his opinions chopped on a platter. "How can you even argue that?"

The fire in her eyes made him want to get to know her more. Her spirited responses intrigued him in a way no woman ever had. It made him want to piss her off just to see her reaction.

"He didn't care about Christmas until the singing disturbed his peace. He just wanted to make the noise stop." Dex shrugged, knowing the casual reply would get her worked up. "I kinda relate to the guy. I used to have this nice, peaceful life where I went to work and came home to the serenity of this house, but then this adorable sexy nurse started ordering me around, and before I even knew it had happened, she replaced my quiet with Christmas carols and the crinkle of ribbons."

"Are you calling me bossy?"

With as much innocence as he could muster, Dex said, "*I* was just telling a story. What meaning *you* derived from it is entirely on you."

"You are calling me bossy!" She stepped up to him and poked him right in the chest. Hard. "I am not bossy."

He laughed, resisting the urge to rub the spot on his chest where she'd just poked him so hard he might have a bruised lung. "Says the woman who barged into my house carrying her body weight in gift wrap while telling me exactly how we are going to spend my night off."

Her eyes narrowed at him. "We talked about—"

She broke off with a squeak when he threw her over his shoulder and carried her back into the living room, where Christmas carols still played from her phone.

"Dexter Henry, you put me down this instant!"

"If we are going to wrap gifts, let's get to it." With a smirk, he set her back on her feet. He faked a bow. "Where do we begin, Taskmaster?"

Grabbing one of the shopping bags sitting by his fireplace, she shoved it against his chest. Anger sparkled in her eyes like he'd hoped it would. His plan was working out just as he'd hoped.

"Start with this one. It's small. Surely you can handle wrapping it."

Again, he laid on the innocent act, nice and thick. "But that's my gift to you. You're not meant to see it until Christmas."

All of the irritation drained from her face. With eyes wide, she stared up at him. "What?"

"You heard me." He flashed her a shy sort of smile when he saw how much the wholesomeness was getting to her. "I can't wrap your gift in front of you."

"When did you…?" She trailed off, eyes filled with wonder that had him curious about when she last had an unexpected gift. "Why would you…?"

"After you left me at the mall, and because you are my girlfriend."

"Fake girlfriend," she corrected.

Shrugging his shoulders, he said softly, "I can't take you home as my girlfriend and not have a gift for you to put under the tree. As you said about your family, my family will also have certain expectations, and believe me, it will not end well for me if I don't put something under the tree for you."

Her eyes were bright and she blinked rapidly as if blinking away unshed tears. "I didn't think to get you anything."

"Then it's a good thing you have a few days before we leave," he teased, trying to lighten the mood. Had he taken things too far with teasing her?

When she didn't smile back, Dex took her hand in his. His touch was warm and welcoming and a million other little things that she should not be thinking of about a man only meant to be her fake boyfriend for a few short weeks. The logical plan would be they'd get through the next few weeks without either of them doing something stupid like falling for the other.

But nothing about the way she felt in that moment was logical.

Her heart beat faster as Dex tugged her closer. The skin-to-skin contact should have been nothing. They were barely holding hands. Should have been… From this close, she got a nice view of the jagged little scar on his chin that she'd always thought was a natural cleft. She wanted to kiss it and—

*Oh, no.*

Her lips could not meet any part of Dex's body, not even the scarred cleft in his chin. Swallowing hard, she took a giant step back from him. Hopefully with some physical distance between them she could get herself under control.

"You know what? I bought myself a new sweater that still has the tags on it," he said. "We can wrap that up as your gift to me. You'll even know that I'll like it and that it fits because I picked it out myself."

Being near him made her crazy. If she wasn't wanting to throw herself at him, she wanted to cry at his thoughtfulness.

This man... He had bought her a gift. Maybe it was part of the ruse to fool his parents, but she couldn't help but be touched by the gesture. It hadn't even occurred to her that she should get him something. And now he added an offer to let her wrap something he'd bought for himself? She wasn't quite sure how to handle that, but one thing for sure was that she couldn't accept that last offer.

"I can't give you a gift you bought yourself after you bought me something. What sort of price range am I spending?" She fought back a sniff. His considerate nature brought her nearly to tears.

"You really don't have to get me anything."

The last dregs of tears dried up with the frustration his non-answer had sparked. She was sprinting through all the emotions tonight. All of them. For so long, she'd refused to allow herself any sentimentality. She kept people—men especially—at arm's length, afraid she'd end up hurt again, but somehow Dex dug his way under her skin and seemed determined to drown her in her own pent-up emotions.

"What price range?" she repeated through clenched teeth.

A weighted silence settled over them, thick and palpable in the room. Their eyes met and the air between them charged with an invisible battle of wills as Lena and Dex sized each other up.

After a few long seconds, Dex broke the stare and Lena did a little internal dance at the win. Dex exhaled his resignation.

"I spent about a hundred bucks on yours. But don't feel obligated to spend that much on me. I know I make significantly more than you, plus you just paid for a cross-country move and a new place."

Dex had no idea that she'd inherited more money than she'd ever spend from her maternal grandfather. She hadn't even heard the words "trust fund" since moving to Tennessee. One of the upsides to living in Nashville, really. She nearly snorted at his concern for her financial status, but stopped it at the last second. The fewer people in Tennessee who knew about her trust fund, the better.

"You want to put this one up to wrap later, then?" She held the small bag out to him with the slightest shake. Lightweight. And it didn't have a noticeable rattle or rustle other than the crinkle of the nondescript white paper bag. It didn't even have a logo on it to identify what store it came from. Curiosity piqued, she tried to run options through her mind as to what the little bag might contain. When he reached for it, she pulled it back out of his reach. "Or maybe I should just take a little peek?"

"Or maybe you should hand it over before I have to take it from you?"

Laughter bubbled out of her at the mischief shining in his eyes. "If you think you are man enough, come get it."

"Is that a dare? You're gonna regret that." Dex grabbed up the spools of ribbon and started pelting her with them.

"Oh, you are going to get it now!" she squealed. The decorative onslaught sparked a war of competitiveness within her. He was going down! Snatching up a roll of wrapping paper, she swung it into his side like a bat. The paper made a lot of noise as it crumpled against his side. "Ha!"

Faster than she could blink, Dex seized the improvised weapon in her hand and pulled her in closer to him. His deep, delicious laughter sent her heart on a jog as he tugged her closer.

And closer.

Dex held tight to the now bent wrapping paper roll with one hand and used the other to brush her hair away from her face. Tucking a lock behind her ear, he cupped her face with his hand.

Lena leaned into his touch. The subtle scent of his cologne wafted over her, its notes reminiscent of the ocean and fresh air. Her eyes fluttered closed as she anticipated his lips on hers.

But then he moved away.

She opened her eyes in confusion.

Dex took another step back, wagging the shopping bag holding her gift back and forth in front of her. He kept walking backward through the open doorway, a wide grin on his face. "I'm going to put this in the bedroom for safekeeping."

"Well played," she grudgingly admitted when he returned. Making her forget she held her own gift took some skill. She'd been too focused on that almost-kiss to notice his actions. The sneak had lifted it right from her distracted and unsuspecting fingers. "I admit defeat. You win that round."

"This is all crinkled up now," he said, picking up the roll of wrapping paper they'd fought over. The red paper was bent nearly in half with creases and wrinkles radiating out from where it had impacted against his body. "I think we need to use this for my brothers' gifts. They won't appreciate pretty paper anyway."

She scoffed. "We can't use wrinkled paper. That's trash now."

"Another Christmas rule?" His brow raised.

"Of course." She gathered up the undamaged supplies and sat down on the floor to get started. Not a single gift had been wrapped. They really needed to get to work if they were going to get everything wrapped in a single evening.

He sat next to her and reached for the pack of bows. "How about you wrap and I'll decorate?"

"I don't think so, Doc. That's not an equal division of labor," she protested as she watched him open the package. "We aren't ready for those yet."

"Shh…" He leaned over and stuck one of the

bows to the top of her head. "I'm wrapping my own present."

"Dex." Her heart barrel-rolled in her chest as the implication of his words crashed hard over her.

"I keep trying to ignore the chemistry between us, but it's hard to do."

Oh, they had chemistry all right. Enough chemistry for six couples and then some, but that didn't mean starting something up would be a good idea. Just chemistry alone wasn't enough to risk a relationship on. Not in her opinion, anyway.

"A meth lab has real chemistry, but it's still hazardous to my health."

Dex's laughter was a laughter that she felt in her own lungs, so deep and joyful that it took her breath away. It erased the concerns and worries she'd had a minute ago and replaced them with a hope that somehow this wouldn't end badly.

"You are a stubborn woman, you know that, Lena Franklin?"

"Says the player who is hitting on me." A giggle rose up and turned into a snort, causing Lena to flush with embarrassment. She dearly loved to laugh, but hated the sounds she made when she did. She argued back, playfully, "It's a lost cause. I'll have you know I have a boy-friend."

"An imaginary one."

"You are not imaginary." Lena laughed until her sides hurt. She had to swipe at a tear trek-king down her cheek. "But that's beside the point. I'm not interested in guys who change girls more than I change my scrubs."

"Fair enough. I'll give you that one." He leaned back against the couch, his pose de-ceivingly relaxed for someone who'd just been shot down hard. "So, what's your story? Who hurt you, Lena? I'm hoping that I'm wrong, but if I was a betting man, I'd put money down that some idiot male screwed up so badly it sent you running across the country to get away from him."

Was she that obvious? Somehow, she'd hoped that her secrets wouldn't follow her, but it didn't seem like she'd been that lucky. Tell-ing Dex about Connor and how much he'd de-ceived her, how gullible and naive she'd been in the search for love, was too much to bear, though.

She tried to change the subject back to some-thing lighter. "I'm going to make you wrap your own presents if you don't behave."

Dex reached over and took her hand in his.

Bending his head, Dex brushed his lips against the back of her wrist, his lips soft and warm against her skin. "I already wrapped the only thing I want."

He stared at her for a moment. The heat radiating up her arm from his touch made her think about things she couldn't have. Things she wouldn't let herself have. Lena swallowed hard. "We should get these presents wrapped."

Coming here tonight might have been a mistake. They'd had such a good time shopping together and she'd learned so much about him in that single day that she'd thought spending more time together would make things easier. But the attraction between them kept things from getting easier. In fact, being near him without giving in to the physical need his touch inspired within her was far harder than she'd anticipated.

"Okay." With one last swipe of his lips over the bare skin of her wrist, Dex released her hand. His intense gaze delved straight into her soul as he said, "I'll back off. For now. What do you want to wrap first?"

# CHAPTER SEVEN

IN THE DAYS since their wrapping paper adventure, something had changed between them. Dex just couldn't put his finger on exactly what. A good change, though, he thought. Lena was relaxing her guard around him, ever so slowly, and opening up with bits and pieces about her past. But whenever he made a move physically, the walls came slamming back into place. Slow and steady was going to be the name of the game with her. He had to ease into this so as not to spook her.

Lena had been all smiles when he'd picked her up for the drive up to Westfield. Her suitcase was nestled in the back of his SUV between his own luggage and the brightly wrapped Christmas presents for his family. Her smile of satisfaction at seeing all the gifts piled in there when he'd put her luggage in had made fiddling with all that ribbon worth it.

"Penny for your thoughts?" Lena asked, tapping him on the arm.

"Just thinking of the other night and how much I enjoyed spending the evening with you."

The colorful paper had been all Lena's idea, but the memory of the evening they spent with rolls of shiny colored paper, curls of ribbon and togetherness would forever be a happy one for him. He hadn't laughed that much in a long time. And Lena softening up to him was a major bonus.

"How can such a gifted surgeon not manage basic gift-wrapping?" She shook her head. Exasperated disbelief filled her voice. "You are hopeless, you know."

"I missed that skills lab," he deadpanned.

The little joke made her laugh. The sound of her laughter was quickly becoming an addiction for him. The more he heard those happy noises, the more he wanted to hear them. She'd told him how she hated her laugh, but for him, it was bright and cheerful, like the mountains around his home covered with fresh snow. There was an imperfect perfection to it and he couldn't get enough.

Dex merged onto the interstate and they began the longest part of the journey home to

Westfield. They had a good four hours on the interstate before they got to Gatlinburg and then would begin the windy mountainous trek to the small town of Westfield, Tennessee.

The excitement of going home was building. There was nothing better than Christmas in the Smoky Mountains. Most of the tourists would be gone after the last of the fall color had faded away for the season, leaving locals and a few random people seeking a quiet country holiday with a view.

He hadn't been home for Christmas in far too long. He'd told his parents he'd had to work because of being the low man on the totem pole. It had always been, "Next year should get better, and I'll come home then." The real truth was that he'd volunteered to work so that he could have a reason to avoid celebrating Christmas. That last Christmas with Jessie had spoiled him on the season.

Then he'd met Lena. Her infectious Christmas spirit had managed to seep into his soul, and he found himself actually looking forward to Christmas this year. He glanced over at the woman in his passenger seat.

Lena shifted around a bit as she found a comfortable position for the long drive. She dug a bag of pretzels out of her purse. "So, what do your parents do? I'm not sure you've ever said."

"My dad is the manager of the town bank and my mom runs the Westfield tourism board. They are pretty involved in all the local issues as a result. You want town gossip, ask my mom. And my dad knows the credit score of everyone in town, probably better than they do. They were so excited when I got into medical school."

"Were?" Lena caught his slip of the tongue and he groaned. He'd revealed more than he'd meant to.

"Are."

"Mmm-hmm." The palm of her hand settled over his forearm. "How much did it disappoint them that you didn't come home and work in Westfield?"

Telling his family that he was not coming back home after med school and residency had been one of the hardest things he'd ever done. His family had always been super close. Tommy had graduated college and moved right back to teach science at the local high school. Jill, his future sister-in-law, had gotten a job at the insurance agency while still in high school, went full-time a minute after graduation and never left town. His youngest brother, Wade, would be right back in Westfield after graduating the next spring with his degree in finance, where his plans were to work at the bank and eventually take over from their dad.

He had been the only one in the family who didn't see a future in the cozy little town. And while his family had never really commented about it, he could see the look in their eyes that said they were hurt he didn't come home to stay, and in the way his mom bit her tongue sometimes when they talked about the future, or his dad stopped midsentence and backtracked.

No matter how much they wanted him home, he couldn't return. It boiled down to one simple fact—there was no place for a general surgeon in his hometown. Westfield didn't even have a proper hospital. It had an emergency room only, no inpatient rooms. It was really for stitches and broken arms. Any actual emergencies were taken to Gatlinburg or Knoxville.

"They thought I would go into family practice and set up shop right on Main Street. But that was never what I wanted." Exhaling slowly, he continued, "From the moment I decided on med school, I wanted to be a surgeon. I put off telling them, though, because I knew how they'd take it."

"I understand going against parental expectations." The pressure her parents had put on her echoed in her words, and he truly believed she did understand.

His parents had hoped he'd come home, yes, but they'd never pressured him to do so. And he knew they never would. However, he didn't think Lena had the same on her end.

"You don't have the best relationship with your parents, do you?"

"What gave it away?" she snarked in reply. "The number of times I've bit your head off for mentioning them or the fact that I hate talking about them?"

"Both?"

A snort came from Lena's direction. "Well, now you know why I wouldn't want to date a guy who is just like my dad, then. I won't become my mother, standing in a man's shadow, lapping up the tiniest scrap of his attention like a sun-starved plant would bask in rays of sunlight. I made that mistake once and refuse to go down that road again."

He looked briefly in her direction. Solid determination masked any other emotion her face might have shown. It told him a lot about who Lena was deep down.

"I don't see much chance of that, as outspoken as you are."

Lena reached over and took his hand in hers. Her fingers tangled with his. "I'm going to take that as a compliment."

"I meant it as one." He rubbed his thumb over her hand. "I told them the truth on how we met, by the way. Well, I said we met at work shortly after you moved to Tennessee."

"That was true. We had that impossibly long surgery with all the peritoneal adhesions about two weeks after I moved here. We stood elbow to elbow for a good eight hours that day."

He remembered that day with perfect clarity. The surgery had taken a good three hours longer than he'd anticipated because of the patient's condition, but he hadn't really minded the extra time because he'd been fascinated by the sharpness of the new nurse at his side who'd known nearly as much about the surgery as he had. She'd impressed him. And when he sought her out later that day, he'd found out that not only was she intelligent, but beautiful as well.

"I asked you out after that surgery."

"Ugh." She scrunched up her nose. "I remember."

"The idea of me asking you out is that distasteful a memory?"

That hurt. He shoved down the initial burst of anger that popped up. His ego was taking a real hit as they rehashed how wrong he'd been about asking Lena out.

"Actually, I was pretty interested." As she continued, her voice grew more confident. "Then I remembered the hospital gossip about you. I can't be one in a line of bed partners for a cocky arrogant surgeon who doesn't care for anything beyond his own needs. Been there, done that, got the heartbreak to prove it."

"Ouch." He wanted to deny her description of him, but there was a grain of truth to her statements. He squeezed her fingers to remind her that she'd taken his hand in hers earlier. "And yet here we are, hand in hand anyways."

"We need to be more comfortable touching each other if we are going to pull this off," she snapped and snatched her hand away. She rubbed it on the thigh of her jeans like he'd contaminated her. "That was your idea, if you remember."

After whatever idiot she'd been involved with had hurt her, prickliness had become her default setting. Each time he pushed too close emotionally, she bristled up like a cactus and went straight into defensive mode.

When he glanced over at her, she was staring out the window and had that stubborn set to her jaw that he was quickly learning meant he wasn't going to win.

"For the record, Lena, I wasn't complaining about holding your hand. In fact, it's been the highlight of my day."

Her cheeks pinked, but she ignored the compliment like he'd expected she would. Trees and exit ramps rolled by as the SUV moved down the interstate. Their conversation trailed off a little, but when he switched on the radio and tuned it to a station playing only Christmas carols, Lena began to hum along.

They passed a sign for a rest area and Lena perked up. "Do you mind if we stop?"

"I could stand to stretch my legs myself." Flipping his blinker on, Dex moved the SUV into the right lane and then onto the exit ramp. He eased to a stop in front of the rest area.

They climbed out of the warm SUV into the brisk December air. A shiver coursed through him and he yanked his zipper up on his jacket to protect himself from the wind.

A woman with two small children—a little girl skipping next to her with a doll in one hand

and a tiny boy in head-to-toe blue who was barely keeping up—came out of the building housing the restrooms. They headed toward the parking lot.

Dex nodded toward them. "Look how adorable they are. In case it comes up, someday I do want to have a couple kids."

"Me too," Lena replied softly. A sadness in her voice when she'd said she wanted children pulled him up short.

But before he could ask her why the thought of having children made her sad, Dex saw the toddler trip and could only watch in horror as the little guy fell face-first onto the concrete walkway.

The thought of how beautiful a baby with Dex's eyes would be sprang to mind, but the image vanished when he suddenly sprinted away from her side. Where was he going in such a rush? She looked in the direction he'd run. The little boy he had just pointed out lay unmoving on the concrete walkway, blood just beginning to pool next to his face.

"He's unconscious," Dex shouted. "Grab the first aid kit from the back of the SUV."

Digging her phone out of her coat pocket, she dialed 911 as she ran back to the car. When the operator answered, Lena quickly gave them what information she could remember. "We are at the rest stop on I-40 between Nashville and Knoxville. I don't know the mile markers. A little boy about two years of age fell face-first onto the concrete walkway here at the rest stop. He's unconscious with some apparent facial injuries based on the amount of blood."

When Lena ran back over, Dex sat on his knees next to the boy. He was trying to explain to the mother why she couldn't pick the child up, because it could worsen his injuries. Despite how much it must be going against her natural instincts, the woman finally just sank to the ground crying. She pulled her daughter into her lap, and her sobs cut sharper than the cold winter wind swirling around them.

"The ambulance is on the way." Lena squatted next to him, opening up the first aid kit and pulling out a roll of gauze.

"What can we do?" His eyes looked tortured as he met her gaze.

"Slow the bleeding." She took the gauze and pressed it to the gaping wound on the child's head. "Here, hold this. We have no equipment. No facilities. All we can do is keep him as warm and as still as possible."

Dex shrugged out of his coat and covered the child with it.

Lena leaned close to the child's chest and listened to his breathing. "Airways seem clear. Breathing is a little rapid." Her fingers felt along the boy's throat. "His pulse is strong and color is still good despite the cold and blood loss."

The little one woke up and started moving, fighting their attempts at helping him and ignoring all their warnings to stay still. He wanted his mother and only barely tolerated them holding the gauze to his wound. It seemed an eternity before they heard the wail of sirens and the ambulance finally pulled up. The paramedics hopped out and hurried over where they took over the boy's care.

Lena and Dex stepped back out of their way.

In moments, the paramedics got the boy loaded into the ambulance, while the boy's mother followed behind with her little girl clinging to her, tears on both their faces.

Dex went to run his hands through his hair as he watched the ambulance drive away, but Lena stopped him.

"You should wash your hands first."

He looked down at his hands, at the blood now drying on his skin. "Good idea."

"Meet you back out here in five?"

He nodded and stomped toward the door with the Men sign hanging overhead.

Lena went the opposite direction to the ladies' room. Random emotions and feelings swirled through her, whipping past her like that icy wind outside. Some fleeting, others lingering, like the desire to see Dex with his own child.

When she was young, she'd dreamed of what it might be like to have a family. To be the mom she'd always wished she'd had, the kind of mom who made messes in the kitchen baking with her kids, and put soccer games before board meetings. And she'd pictured the father of those children as the kind of dad who would build forts and have snowball fights and teach his kids to fix things, not dismiss them to play another round of golf.

Then she'd grown up and babies had become a "someday" thought for her, pushed off even more by the realization that a family meant trusting someone enough to risk a pregnancy. She'd almost considered it with Connor, but then he'd shown his true colors and she'd locked even the hope of ever having a child away in that "never gonna happen" box. But today, seeing the tender way Dex cared for

that little boy had kicked the hint of wondering about what his children might look like into a full-blown need to mother the man's children.

After splashing some water on her face, she looked up at her reflection in the mirror. "Pull yourself together. You need to calm down before you go back out there and jump him in the parking lot." She took several deep breaths and tried to put the idea of seeing Dex holding their child out of her mind.

She walked outside, still trying to talk herself out of creating those imaginary babies right then and there. They would make beautiful babies, but she and Dex were so not to that point. She was barely tolerating a fake relationship. She didn't trust him enough to go on a real date. Something was clearly wrong with her given her current line of thought.

Dex hadn't noticed her yet. She walked behind him, a few paces back, and the tight fit of his shirt across his shoulders and the snug way his jeans molded to his backside did not help her clear her mind.

*Why would that thought not go away?*

Dex picked up his jacket from the ground where it had been tossed aside by the paramedics. He shook it and bits of dirt and dust flew off it, floating away on the crisp breeze.

Lena stopped next to him, nodding toward the bloodstained jacket in his hands. "Pretty sure that's ruined."

He shrugged. "Maybe. Have to take it to the dry cleaner in the morning and see if they can do anything with it. I'm just glad it looks like the little guy will be okay. He had me worried."

"Me too." She quickly stuffed the packets of medication she'd thrown out of the way while looking for gauze back into the first aid kit. She rolled the loose unused gauze into a ball to toss in the trash. "You'll need to refill this soon. The rest of that gauze is unusable thanks to this wind." She closed the plastic container and looked up at him carefully. "Are you okay to drive?"

With a nod, he held a hand out to her. "Guess we need to get moving after our non-rest stop, don't we? It's going to be late by the time we get to Westfield now as it is."

They walked back to his SUV hand in hand. He tossed his jacket into the back before taking the first aid kit from her and placing it inside. Closing the back, he guided her around to the passenger side and opened her door. She was still getting used to the idea that he wanted to open doors for her. But it was another thing she had found that she really liked about Dexter Henry.

"You were amazing out there. I was floundering, trying unsuccessfully to determine where to start outside of a sterile operating room. And you...you just stepped right up and took charge." He brushed a strand of hair back away from her face. "I haven't been this much in awe of someone's medical skills since my first day of medical school."

His admiration sparked a fresh wave of interest in him. It had been a long time since anyone had given her such genuine, heartfelt praise and it felt really, really good. Before she could second-guess the impulse, she moved against him and wrapped her arms around his neck. Tugging his head down to hers, she rose up on tiptoe and pressed her lips to his.

She might have initiated the kiss, but Dex controlled it. His lips moved over hers with a barely reined-in passion. His arms worked their way beneath her coat and behind her back. He held her close, his touch gentle but firm. The kiss held a realness, a promise of something yet to come. Any hint of the relationship being fake flew away on the wind for the duration of their embrace.

When he broke the kiss, they stared at each

other, silent for a moment. His breath warmed her cheek. Her hand rested on his throat and his pulse beat beneath her fingers, rapid and strong.

"Why did you do that?" he asked. "And that's so not a complaint."

"I thought we should have our first kiss before we had to potentially kiss in front of your family." A completely made-up answer slipped from her lips because she couldn't—wouldn't—admit to him that she'd been thinking about having his babies or that his compliments had been enough for her to throw caution to the wind for a brief moment. That would go over well, wouldn't it? *Sorry, I'm scared to date you but I can't wait to see how adorable our children would be.* He'd call her a lunatic.

"One hell of a first kiss."

That was an understatement if she'd ever heard one. She'd known they had a strong physical attraction and she'd still been totally unprepared for the intensity of his lips pressed against her own. Her racing heart served as proof of that, still pounding against her ribs.

He nuzzled against her throat. "How about a second? Wouldn't want to look like amateurs, would we?"

Before she could formulate a coherent response, his lips were on hers. His tongue asked for access and then delved into her mouth when she parted her lips in permission. He wasn't just kissing her, he was savoring her.

When they broke apart for the second time, he rested his forehead against hers while they both gasped for air. The chemistry between them had been exactly why Lena had been hesitant to get involved with Dex. Nothing short of magical, his kiss made her think stupid thoughts. Things a rational woman shouldn't be thinking. Long-term, family planning, scary sorts of things.

She swallowed hard, needing to put some distance between them and regain her perspective. "We should go before your mama sends out a search party."

Dex groaned and stepped back. "Way to kill the mood, Lena."

The mood had not been killed for her. But she was trying her best to murder it because Dexter Henry was a temptation she no longer wanted to resist.

*No!*

She had to resist. This relationship was meant to be fake. Falling into anything with

Dex would only lead to heartache. No lust, no beds, and definitely no love.

She climbed into the SUV and leaned her head back into the seat. This thing was spiraling out of her control and she had no idea how to stop it now. She had to remind him that this was fake and she had to keep her distance. Simple as that.

A moment later, Dex was in the driver's seat next to her and they were back on the interstate heading to his hometown. Dex remained quiet as he maneuvered the SUV through the holiday traffic.

As the mile markers flew past, Lena tried to pull herself together. She just needed to get through the next two weeks and then they'd be back in Nashville, back to their normal lives, where they could go back to only seeing each other at the hospital and only talking about patients. That had always been the plan. A few kisses didn't change that.

Kissing Dex was definitely at the top of things that she should have never done, but couldn't bring herself to regret. She'd moved to Tennessee for a fresh start, though, and she wasn't going to mess that up because of a surgeon with enough passion in his kiss to make her knees weak. She just needed to make it through the holidays without falling for Dex.

Even if that seemed like an impossible task at the moment.

"We're here." Dex pulled to a stop in front of his parents' house just before midnight. Christmas lights and decor covered the log cabin that nestled into the edge of the forest. The eaves were outlined in colorful lights, while white lights outlined the shape of reindeer and a sleigh next to the sidewalk. The holiday adornment gave it a very festive feel.

As they walked up the sidewalk to the front door, she grabbed his hand and tugged him to a stop. The need to put them back on level ground overwhelmed her. "Despite how intense those kisses were, we need to remember that this is fake."

"Is it though?" His thumb rubbed temptingly along the back of her hand.

"It has to be," she said with a conviction she didn't quite feel anymore. "We can't get too carried away and forget that this is all for show."

His stare sliced straight to her soul. The hint of a grin on his lips said he didn't believe her. "If you say so."

"I do." She'd told him how things needed

to be. She'd just keep her distance as much as possible and that way she'd be sure to get through this unscathed. Lena told herself these things even if she wasn't quite sure that she even believed them.

When the door opened, she came face-to-face with Dex's mother for the first time. Lena put a smile on her lips as they reached the top of the steps. She could only hope her smile didn't look as fake as she felt.

# CHAPTER EIGHT

"DEXTER, GET OVER HERE!"

"Hey, Mama," Dex said, dropping his suit-case as soon as he reached the porch so that he could give his mom a hug. "What are you still doing up? We could have let ourselves in."

"Oh, you know I couldn't sleep 'til I knew you were home safe."

When his mom pulled him into a warm hug, his guilt spiked. He had to spend the next week lying to his parents. As much as he'd wanted to see his parents, he'd been hoping that their late arrival would buy him a few more hours free of lying. He'd even briefly entertained the thought of faking an emergency and heading back to Nashville before his parents woke up in the morning, of letting them see Lena for only a moment before disappearing back to Nashville with her and making an excuse for why she didn't make it back for the wedding.

"Where on earth is your coat? It's freezing

out here." His mom released her hold on him enough to back up to arm's length. She held on to his biceps and looked him over critically. He could almost see the calculations in her mind as she examined him. "Are you eating enough? You look too skinny."

Lena laughed from beside him and he caught the note of disbelief. With a single brow raised, he glanced over at her in question.

She brushed his question off with a wave of her hand. "It's nothing."

"It's not nothing. I heard that tone."

Rolling her eyes at him, she said, "Laughs don't have tones, Dex."

"Yours do," he argued.

Lena sighed, but her jaw wasn't set in stubborn refusal. If he had to put an emotion on her expression, he'd say she was a little sad.

"It's just… Well, your mom worries that you are too skinny. Next week mine will be lecturing me about how I need to watch my waistline and insisting that I must be eating too much. She'll probably even suggest I go in for a consult about liposuction."

"Hmmph." His mom reached out and pulled Lena toward her. "Come over here in the light where I can see you better." Mrs. Henry clicked her tongue, her head shaking as she did. "Why, you aren't as big as a minute, and if your mama can't see how beautiful you are then she needs to get her eyes checked."

Lena's shocked expression made his heart hurt. She seemed genuinely surprised that his mom thought she was beautiful. He didn't think she had a clue just how gorgeous she was. If only she could see herself the way he saw her.

His mom put her arm around Lena and ushered her toward the door. "Now you two get in here out of the cold before you freeze solid and I turn you into lawn ornaments for the rest of the winter. I made some chili earlier and I can heat you some right up." She looked over her shoulder at him, concern darkening her eyes. "You need something warm in you after being out in that cold, and without a coat. For such a smart boy, I wonder about your common sense some days, Dexter. You're gonna catch your death being out in this wind without even a sweater on."

Like most of the single-family homes in Westfield and the greater Gatlinburg area, his parents' home was a rustic log cabin. Even the interior was filled with dark wood, from the walls down to the hardwood floors. Being more at home on a hiking trail than in a fancy restaurant meant that his mom didn't care for frills and lace, though. No, her style was more handmade quilts, cozy plaids and soft blankets. This house he'd grown up in was a cozy family home, but it wouldn't win any decorating awards. Dex was sure it wasn't what Lena was used to, but hopefully she'd feel at home here.

"Wow," Lena said as she took her coat off in the living room. She spun in a slow circle and looked around. "This place is amazing. It reminds me of a cabin we rented in Aspen one year when my parents wanted to ski for Christmas, but with far less dead animals hanging on the walls. Thankfully. All those eyes staring down at you is creepy."

His mom reached out and squeezed Lena's hand in commiseration. "Oh, I'm right there with you on that, honey, and I promise you, there are none of God's creatures preserved in an unnatural state under this roof. Not while I'm alive. Let me get you all that chili."

"You ski?" Dex asked Lena while his mom walked away. Lena didn't seem like the skiing type to him, so hearing that she'd spent a Christmas on the slopes in Aspen was a surprise.

"Not at all." Lena shook her head and gave a little laugh, almost a snort. "*They* spent the week on the slopes. My much older nanny hated the cold, however, so she and I spent a lot of time at the clubhouse having hot chocolate and working jigsaw puzzles."

Even though she laughed, it sounded forced and pain laced her words. It gave him more insight into her relationship with her parents and helped explain why they weren't close. What sort of parents ditched their only child at Christmas? His heart hurt as he envisioned a tiny Lena hanging out at the clubhouse with an old lady, her face pressed against the window watching while the other kids were out on the slopes with their parents, or worse, watching her parents ski away without a backward glance.

"Was that a typical Christmas for you then?" he asked, taking her hand and pulling her over to the couch.

She sank down next to him, leaning into his side, and he felt more than heard the sadness in her exhalation. "Being alone with the nanny somewhere adjacent to where my parents did something fun? Yes, that was a traditional Christmas for us. I'd be decked out in a fancy dress and paraded out whenever they wanted to prove they were parents. Sometimes I'd be forced to perform for them and their friends. But otherwise they did their thing while I stayed behind with the nanny."

Dex swallowed hard. "Perform?" he asked hesitantly. Given that she was finally opening up, he didn't want her to shut down again.

"Piano, sing, one year they put me in tap dance lessons before they realized I was far too clumsy to ever succeed at that." She smiled at him, a pitiful little grimace, really, that didn't reach her eyes. "It nearly turned me off Christmas entirely."

He gaped at her, dumbfounded. "You love Christmas so much, though."

"Now I do." Lena shrugged and pulled one of the throw pillows into her lap. She fidgeted with the decorative trim around its edge. "Our house never decorated for Christmas when I was growing up because it wasn't like we were going to be home, so when I moved out on my own, the first year I went all out as a bit of rebellion, but then... Then going all out for Christmas became *my* tradition, ya know? Even if I'm alone, it's something that no one can take from me. While a lot of things are more fun with someone else, it's still nice to decorate a tree, or build a gingerbread house, or go look at Christmas lights."

It hadn't taken him long to realize that Lena

isolated herself because connecting with people scared her. She wasn't really antisocial; she was anti getting hurt. And who could blame her for that after the upbringing she'd had? Everything he learned about her past made him think that her icy exterior was a veneer designed to protect her from the pain of involvement. He saw it in the hot-cold way she reacted to him. She warmed up until she realized how much she was letting him in, and then she took a step back to put that distance between them that would protect her heart.

Maybe he recognized it so easily because in a lot of ways he was just like her. He hadn't retreated within himself to the extent Lena had, but he guarded his emotional interactions with others and didn't freely allow people close because he knew what it felt like to have his heart shattered until he didn't recognize himself anymore. He knew the pain of loss.

But Lena had such a caring heart and truly beautiful soul that he hated to see her withdrawing from everyone like she had.

Squeezing her tight, Dex pressed a kiss to the top of her head. "New rule of Christmas, no more spending it alone."

Lena swiped at a tear trailing down her

cheek, but she smiled at him through her tears. "You said there were no rules to Christmas."

He rubbed his thumb over the errant tear she'd missed. "Your rules are growing on me."

With Dex so close, still cupping her cheek gently, his hand warm and perfect against her skin, Lena did the only thing she could do. She leaned forward and pressed her lips to his. Unlike the kisses at the rest stop that were hungry and carried a sort of desperation, this kiss was gentle and comforting.

His lips moved over hers slowly, sensually. Each movement a caress. His thumb grazed her cheekbone as he moved it over her skin, mimicking the movements of his lips.

Lena sighed as she relaxed into his embrace.

A throat clearing in the doorway pulled them apart and Lena's cheeks heated. She pressed her face into Dex's shoulder, feeling like she could die of embarrassment, while he merely laughed.

"It's not funny," she whispered, which only seemed to make him laugh harder. "What's your mom going to think of me?"

His mom hadn't been gone but long enough to heat up a couple bowls of chili and came back to them practically all over each other.

They weren't setting themselves up for his mom to like her at all.

With her embarrassment now complete, Lena smiled shyly over at Dex's mom. "Hello," she said, without knowing what else to say.

*This is going well*, she thought sarcastically.

"I brought the two of you some chili. The corn bread's gone, but I have some saltines that'll be near as good." Dex's mother set a loaded silver tray on the coffee table in front of them. She raised a brow at Dex in censure. "I didn't expect to find the two of you making out like teenagers when I came back."

Lena cringed. Exactly what she'd been afraid of…his mom hated her and they hadn't been here an hour. Less than an hour had to be a new record.

Dex handled his mother in a way Lena would never have attempted—with a joke. "Well, you did say for me to come inside and warm up. What better way is there to warm up than in the arms of a beautiful woman?"

"Mmm-hmm…" Mrs. Henry shook her head at them, but there was a hint of a smile on her face. "Eat your chili while its hot. Dexter, you know where to find your room. The two of you keep it down, though. Your aunt Peggy is asleep in Tommy's room next door. And if your brother gets too loud with those video games, you remind him I said he better not wake anyone up cussing at some cartoon man on the television just because the poor thing ran off a cliff like he was told."

Lena suppressed a snicker. She doubted either of Dex's brothers played any sort of game that involved running a cartoon character off a cliff. Not at their ages.

Then a stressful realization dawned on her. His mother had implied they were sharing a room. That was not in the plans.

Not at all.

She couldn't share a room—or a bed—with Dex. She swallowed hard. She just *couldn't*. Not if she wanted to make it through this unscathed. He'd assured her there was no need for a hotel room because his parents had a spare room. Had he planned this all along?

Whispering to Dex, Lena asked, "I don't suppose your room has two beds in it, does it?"

He gave his head one swift shake in the negative.

"Eat now." His mother tapped on the tray. "I'm going to bed and will see the two of you in the morning. That's soon enough for me to get to know this lovely girl you've brought home." She stood and rounded the couch to stand behind them. She enclosed them both in a loose hug, kissing Dex on the top of the head. "Don't stay up too late."

Lena watched as the older woman walked toward the back of the house. Lights flicked off until they were left in only the light of a lamp next to the couch and the light above the stairs across from them.

"I had no idea Aunt Peggy would be here or I'd have rented us a place nearby. There aren't any hotels in Westfield, but there are quite a few rental cabins. The last I'd heard, Aunt Peggy wasn't coming in for the wedding." Dex leaned forward and grabbed his bowl of chili. "I'll sleep down here on the couch. It'll be fine for tonight and we will see tomorrow about getting a rental for the rest of the week."

"What will your mom say?"

"Probably think we had a fight after she went to bed." Dex shrugged. "And she'll probably get her feelings hurt by us getting a rental, but she'll get over it. Eventually."

Lena closed her eyes and tried to wrap her mind around what the best course of action would be. If he slept down here, that left her sleeping in his bed alone. And the idea of upsetting his mother did not sit well with her. "I don't want her to think we are fighting, especially not on the first day we're here. And how would it look if we had a fight just minutes after she walked in on us kissing?"

"It would make us breaking up next month more realistic." Lifting one shoulder in a half-hearted shrug, Dex added, "Besides that, our options are pretty limited. I either sleep down here or I sleep with you."

"I guess you are sleeping with me tonight, then. It doesn't feel right to take your bed and kick you to the couch."

"I'd be more than happy to share a bed with you, Lena."

The passion behind those words made it far more than a simple tease. Ducking her head to hide the blush she felt creeping up her cheeks, Lena tried to put the idea of sharing a bed out of her mind and focused her thoughts instead on what he said about a fight making their breakup more realistic.

"We can stage a fight later this week, maybe. I don't want her thinking I'm totally wrong for you from day one and making the entire week miserable and tense. We'll have enough of that with my family, trust me."

"You don't want her to think you don't like her chili either." He waved his spoon at her bowl still sitting on the tray untouched. "Eat."

Lena picked up the bowl of chili. Steam no longer rose from the surface, but warmth flooded her fingers from the heated stoneware. The heady aroma of peppers and spices wafted up from the surface. "It smells good."

"Tastes even better."

She dipped her spoon in and hazarded a taste. "Ooh, that's spicy." She blinked rapidly as her eyes began watering. Wow. It was hotter than she'd expected.

"It's character-building. Put some crackers in it. That'll tone it down, city girl."

Lena dipped the saltine in the spicy chili and had to admit that Dex was right. The cracker calmed the heat down enough that she could tolerate it.

"What does me being a city girl have to do with thinking this chili is too spicy?" she asked as she tried to let some of the heat dissipate off her tongue.

Dex tucked a lock of her hair behind her ear and smiled at her, the dim light of the room throwing part of his face into shadow and making it hard to read his expression. "Not a thing. But you told me I can't call you honey anymore, so I'm trying to honor that."

"What's wrong with my name?"

"Not a thing."

He laid his hand on her jeans-clad thigh, and the heat from his palm sent her heart racing like she'd climbed the mountainous road into Westfield on foot instead of in the passenger seat of an SUV. She swallowed hard when he leaned close. Her breath caught in anticipation that he might kiss her again.

"You gonna eat the rest of that chili?"

"Oh, you…" She shoved the bowl into his broad chest. "You have it. I don't think I can take any more anyway. My eyes are boiling as it is."

With her nerves in an uproar at Dex's closeness, Lena tried to get a handle on her emotions and thoughts while he finished off the second bowl of chili. Over the last few hours, she and Dex had moved into dangerous territory for a fake relationship. She'd anticipated having to kiss him. After all, their families were meant to think they were serious enough to be meeting the family, and that meant the expectation of at least a low level of PDA. She'd even braced herself for the desire that washed over her at every touch of his hand.

But the way he placed his hand on the small of her back when he walked next to her? Or how those little lines appeared and crinkled just so at the corners of his eyes when he laughed? And most of all, the way his expression softened sometimes when he looked at her?

Those things she hadn't been ready for.

He tapped her on the nose. "Lost in thought?"

"Hmm…" Her cheeks heated with embarrassment at being caught staring at him. Hopefully in the dimly lit room he wouldn't be able to see the color surely darkening up her cheeks. "Just tired. It's been a long day."

"That it has. Wait here. I'll stick these bowls in the dishwasher and then we can get to bed."

Lena tried to relax while she waited, but the knowledge that in just a few short moments she'd be in the same bed as Dex had her too keyed up to manage it. Anticipation and dread warred within her and she wasn't quite sure which would win out in the end.

He walked back in and held out his hand. When he spoke, his words were loaded with innuendo and her heart beat so loud in her ears that it nearly drowned him out.

"Come on, city girl, let me take you to bed."

# CHAPTER NINE

DEX NOTICED THE momentary panic in Lena's eyes before a wary desire moved in. Cautious interest he could deal with. Fear, not so much. He didn't want her to be afraid of him. She had to come to him willingly.

"You don't have to be afraid of me, Lena," he said with his hand still outstretched. He waited to see if she was going to take that step and put her hand in his. To see if she trusted him enough to move forward with him in this way.

After a moment where she nibbled her lips and he nearly closed the distance himself, Lena swallowed hard. But her voice was rock solid when she said, "I'm not afraid of you, Dexter Henry." She stepped away from him to grab her bag, and what she said next he didn't think she meant him to hear.

But he thought he heard her say, "I'm afraid of my reactions to you."

"I'm so tired I could sleep on these stairs, how 'bout you?"

"Exhausted." She looked up the steep stairs, slung her bag over her shoulder and sighed. "A hotel would have had a bellhop to carry our bags up for us."

"I can get it for you, if you need me," he offered.

"No, I can do it. You know, if we stay at my parents' like my mother wants, they have 'Robert,' who will carry them up for us." She used her fingers to make quotations around the name.

"Robert?" he asked, making air quotes like she had. "Why would you put air quotes around a person's name?"

Her expression was one of long suffering mingled with annoyed disbelief. It intrigued him how much she could say in a single glance. Her face expressed more emotions than people he knew. Or maybe he was just so intrigued by her that even her microexpressions couldn't slip past his scrutiny? He packed that last thought away for later examination.

"Because our butler's real name is usually not Robert. My mother just can't be bothered to learn any new names, so when someone gets hired there, they take on the mantle of Robert."

"I'm sorry, what?" Surely he had misunderstood what she'd just said. No one could be so egotistical as to rename their employees, could they?

"All our butlers are named Robert now, regardless of what their given name is." She shrugged. "Please don't judge me on this. I have no say in what my parents do."

"Wow. Just…wow."

"I know." She waved toward the stairs. "Can we…?"

"Oh, right." He took her bag from her hand. "I'll carry this. Consider me your own personal Robert."

She snorted. "I'm never going to live this one down, am I?"

"Probably not, city girl," he called over his shoulder as he led the way up the stairs. He walked into his childhood bedroom and dropped the suitcases at the foot of the bed. Looking around, he tried to see if anything too embarrassing still lingered in here. He hadn't stayed with his parents in years, after all, and never with a woman he cared about impressing. Nothing jumped out at first glance, at least.

Lena leaned against the open door frame.

"Okay, so we need to set some ground rules before we get in that bed."

"Shh…" Dex pointed quickly toward the wall on his left. With his voice barely above a whisper, he continued, "You would think with ten-inch-thick log walls you'd have some privacy, but sound carries in this place like you were standing next to each other. The only privacy in this house is visual."

How sound carried in this cabin was his least favorite thing about his childhood home. His mom had always known exactly what kind of mischief he was up to practically before he started because she could hear everything he did. Everything he said.

Maybe even what he thought.

"Really?" She wrinkled her nose up and stared at the wall separating his room from the room where his aunt slept. "Strike log cabins off my list of future dream homes, then."

"For real." He rolled his eyes. He'd made that determination himself years ago. "And when I was a kid, my parents had the room next door. They didn't build the addition downstairs until I was in high school."

"Lovely."

Shaking his head at her, he said, "That's a word someone would use who was not regularly subjected to hearing just how much their parents still loved each other."

"That would imply that said person's parents actually ever loved each other." Wrapping her arms around herself, she grimaced. "I told you that love didn't factor into my parents' decisions. Pretty sure my parents are only together because they each had something to offer to the other. My mother came from old money. But my dad had the hotshot career and the more varied social connections that my mother desired. And after thirty years together, neither is willing to admit defeat or suffer the societal downturn that a divorce would entail."

"Surely they loved each other at some point. They had you, after all."

"No, they needed an heir to parade about as proof they were really married." The melancholy etched on her face cut straight to the depths of his soul. "I happened to be who they got stuck with. Both would have preferred a son."

Dex moved in front of her and tugged her into his arms. He wanted to soothe away her sadness and give her some happy memories. And that vulnerability in her gaze made him want to do whatever it took to protect her. He stiffened at that thought and rolled the idea around in his head. Protect her? Where did that come from? And why did it feel so natural?

"Dex, this isn't a good idea."

"I told you before, I'm a big boy and I know what *no* means."

Even though his voice was a low whisper, the hurt and frustration slammed into her like a wave pounding at the sand. This man had her emotional state sitting on a fault line that spanned her already fragile heart. She needed time to stabilize it before anymore seismic activity worsened it. But at the same time, if she continually hurt him with her actions, then she was no better than her father.

"When I'm tired, my emotions run closer to the surface, and I don't want to subject you to another potential meltdown," she admitted.

He took a step back and slid his hands down her arms, linking his fingers with hers. His voice was barely audible. "You know I'd never want to cause you pain, right? I know I have a bit of a reputation—"

"A bit?" she scoffed, interrupting him. "According to hospital gossip, you've slept with half the female staff under forty."

"Not even close. But even if I had, what's

wrong with two consenting adults finding a few moments of pleasure with one another?"

"A few moments, huh?" She leaned closer, her lips grazing his ear. "Never pegged you for a two-punch chump."

The speed with which he moved surprised her and the next thing she knew, Dex had her pinned to the wall. His teeth nipped at her earlobe with a sharp warning. "If you don't want to find out about my skills in the bedroom, then don't tease."

In the span of a breath, the dynamic between them shifted from something awkward that still held a layer of falsehood to something far deeper. Swallowing hard, Lena put her hands up on his shoulders to push him away—which was the responsible thing to do, of course—but just as she did, he nuzzled his way down her throat, and the thought of rejecting his advances fled.

"Dex…"

"You want me to kiss you, don't you?"

"Mmm-hmm." She didn't trust her words in that moment. But yes, she wanted him to kiss her. More than she'd ever wanted anyone to kiss her.

"Well, well, well, what have we here?"

"Wade!" Dex spun around. "You saw nothing. You heard nothing. And if you tattle on me, then I'm going to hit you so hard you'll have a dent for a week."

"Dex, if you hit him that hard you'll break your hand and you might not be able to cut anymore. I've seen what happens when surgeons can't operate anymore. I don't want to live through that again." She shivered, despite the heat lingering from Dex's touch. "Maybe kick him instead?"

When her father had lost the full use of his hand after a car accident, their lives had been nearly destroyed by the man's own self-pity. Once he'd moved past the initial depression, he'd thrown all his energy into trying to mold Lena into his replacement. But she'd never been interested in plastic surgery. She'd disappointed him when instead of pre-med she'd chosen nursing. It was only after he'd accepted the medical director position that things had slowly got back to normal, where he'd mostly ignored her and worked constantly again.

"Lena, this is Wade, my youngest brother." Dex waved a hand in Wade's general direction, then waved toward her. "Annoying baby brother, this is my girlfriend, Lena."

Her heart skipped a beat as her referred to her as his girlfriend again. She hadn't quite solved the mystery of why her body liked that term so much. Was it the way the word rolled off his tongue in that sexy Southern accent he tried so hard to squash?

Or, and she hated to even admit this to herself, was it because Dex was the first man ever to make her feel valued? And he did it so effortlessly.

"Hello," she said, flashing a smile at Wade. So that's what Dex had looked like in college.

Wade had the same dark hair and the same broad shoulders, but there was something about him that seemed lesser. Maybe a lack of maturity? She couldn't quite put her finger on it.

Dex and Wade started talking and she moved into the bedroom without either of them being aware. They moved down the hallway into another room, their quiet conversation carrying just barely through the space.

She sighed when she sank down on the bed. Flopping back, she closed her eyes against the burn of tears. Having Dex's brother interrupt was frustrating, of course, but it had also kept them from potentially taking things a step too far. A step they weren't really prepared to take.

At least with Dex down the hall catching up with his brother—and judging from the occasional laughter and unending conversation, he might be a while—she had the room to herself for the moment. And that was a relief.

Sitting back up, she went into the attached bath and got ready for bed. Dex was still down the hall when she flipped off the lights and climbed under the covers. If they were both lucky, she'd be sound asleep by the time he had finished reminiscing with his brother. Because if she was awake, they might find themselves in a situation that didn't get interrupted.

And she wasn't sure if that would be a good thing or not.

# CHAPTER TEN

THE ALLURING AROMA of coffee tickled at his awareness. Dex rolled over and reached for Lena, his hand coming up empty, and the sheets on the other side of the bed were cold.

"Lena?" He sat up, rubbing at his eyes.

With the bathroom door standing open, he could be sure she wasn't in the en suite. She'd fallen asleep while he and his brother had caught up. He'd been tempted to wake her up and finish what they'd started before Wade's interruption, but she'd looked so peaceful that he'd let her sleep.

She'd been in his arms when he'd fallen asleep. Now where the heck was she?

A few minutes later, after he'd got dressed, he made his way down the stairs. Soft feminine laughter carried through the cabin from the kitchen. He stopped in the doorway to see what he was walking into.

Lena stood in the kitchen wrapped in one of

his mother's oversized aprons, her hair piled loosely on top of her head. She focused on a bowl of batter before her on the island countertop. Concentration wrinkled her forehead as she scrutinized the batter. "Is it meant to be so lumpy?"

"You never made pancakes before?" Dex asked in disbelief.

Lena waved a whisk with clumps of flour clinging to it in his direction. "Hush, you. I told you I don't know how to cook much."

"Does 'Robert' make your pancakes, then?"

She rolled her eyes at him. "Butlers do not cook. Robert would be insulted if asked to make pancakes. He could be sent to ask Chef to do so, however."

"You have a butler?" his mom asked with disbelief. "Stir that batter a little more. It shouldn't be quite that lumpy, but a few lumps are okay."

Lena stirred the batter slowly and carefully, her attention focused on it. "My parents have a butler, not me. They have a butler, a chef, a housekeeper and a gardener. Robert, the butler, is in charge of the others as well as being my father's personal assistant. When I was younger, they had my nanny as well."

"Your parents must be busy people." His

mom tried to be diplomatic, but he could see on her face how she really felt. She'd never tell Lena that she thought people with that many servants were ridiculous, because she wouldn't want to hurt Lena's feelings. But they'd had a lot of arguments just getting his mom to accept help with even occasional housekeeping. She was old-fashioned and believed a woman should take care of her own home and family.

"You won't hurt it if you stir a little more vigorously. Give it a good stir." Dex stepped closer and put his hand over Lena's.

"Busy? Sure." Lena's sigh reached deep and held frustration as she came back to his mom's question. "My father had his practice and later the hospital to run. Mother had her charities."

"And what did you have?" Dex questioned, noticing she'd left herself out of that explanation. He wrapped his arms around Lena from behind and pressed a soft kiss to the side of her throat. There was a naturalness to the move that settled over him. Holding Lena in his arms felt right.

"Paralyzing self-doubt, endless anxiety and so much fear of commitment that I could be my own Halloween attraction?" Lena gave him a raw, honest answer, deeper than she meant to give if the blush that soared up into her cheeks was any indication. "Forget I said that, please," she murmured.

How could he forget what she said when she'd just given him so much insight into her history? He held her closer. "That's why you turned me down at first, isn't it?"

"She did what?" his mom interrupted, sounding really surprised. "Turned you down? When?"

"Shh…" He shushed his mom. "Lena and I have moved past it, so don't think on it."

Lena sighed and leaned back against his chest. "After surgery that day, when we'd spent all that time side by side, and just talking, you know, I got to thinking, maybe I could get lucky and find someone who would really see me and want to be with me. Not because of who I was related to, or the connections I could offer them, but the real me. But, well, I let the gossip get into my head. So, yes, my parents were part of why I turned you down, but I let other people convince me that you were like *him* and I couldn't—"

Dex spun her around. "I'd never—"

Lena cut him off with a sound. He pressed his lips shut and waited for her to finish her thoughts.

"I couldn't risk it. Not 'til I got to know you

better. And the more I get to know you, the more I realized that the only thing you have in common with my father and Connor is that you are all surgeons." Lena reached up and cupped his cheek. "I've also realized that I'm going to have to accept the loss on these pancakes. I think I'll go get a shower now."

He watched as Lena took the apron off. She folded it neatly and placed it on the island before heading upstairs.

With a deep sigh, he sank down onto a stool.

"Trouble in paradise?" his mom asked. She nodded in the direction of the stairs. "I'm having a hard time getting a feel on her. She flutters from friendly to frosty faster than a honeybee in your Nana's flower garden."

He shrugged. "I'm hungry. You got any pancakes made?"

"You just gonna ignore my question?" Her brow rose as she looked him over, scrutinizing his face while waiting for him to answer. Ignoring her was never an option. She'd hound him until she got the answers she wanted out of pure stubbornness.

"No, ma'am, I'm not ignoring you. I was just trying to think of the right way to phrase what I need to say." The need to protect Lena rose up again. He wanted to defend her to his mom, but he didn't want to overshare something Lena might have said in confidence either.

"How many pancakes you want?" His mom lifted the cover on the cake plate where she'd stacked up the pancakes she'd made.

"Three's good. Thanks." He took the plate of pancakes offered. "Lena had a far different upbringing than I did. She wants to be friendly, really, she does. She's not used to sharing feelings and such like she just did. When she does, and she realizes how much she shared, it scares her. Then she frosts over and retreats. Give her a little time and she'll be right back down here with a smile."

"Oh, that poor girl." His mom looked toward the stairs. He recognized that look—Lena just became his mom's new project. "Well, we will make her fit in here and she'll know she can trust us."

"It would mean the world to me if you did." He popped a bite of pancake in his mouth, chewing slowly while he considered the implications behind that. Those agreed-upon boundaries were starting to get a little fuzzy for him and he wasn't sure how he felt about that. If she wasn't starting to feel the same, he could be setting himself up for a whole world of heartache.

Since his disastrous engagement, he'd kept his relationships short and sweet. A few weeks, maybe a month, max, and then they parted ways. He didn't stick around long enough for there to be drama. He'd already invested more time in getting to know Lena than he had in his last three relationships. And yet, he didn't regret a moment of it.

"Does Lena make you happy?" his mom asked, rubbing his back.

"She does. I can see a real future with her."

"Oh!" She nearly squealed and pulled him into a big, tight hug. "You have no idea how long I have been waiting to hear you say that! It does this old heart good to hear that."

Saying that had maybe taken this fake relationship a step too far toward real. He had never been good at lying to his mother. She'd always seen through any charade he'd attempted and had known his every transgression as a child almost before he'd done it. How he would make it through the next few days without spilling his guts and admitting the truth, he wasn't quite sure. But was he really lying to her this time?

That was the real question, wasn't it?

"While Lena's upstairs, I wanted to ask…" His mother paused for dramatic effect.

And his heart stopped. The pancakes he'd just eaten sat heavy in his stomach, a gluttonous brick weighing him down. He pushed away his half-finished breakfast, having suddenly lost his appetite. She always saved "the pause" for when she was about to call him out for the transgression he'd thought he'd gotten by with.

"How are you really feeling about Jessie's return?"

"Jessie?" His heart started up again with an odd lurch. She wanted to talk about Jessie? "I…uh… Well, I'm sure Ray and Mary will be happy to have her home."

He'd always liked Jessie's folks. They'd been like a second set of parents to him when he'd been with their daughter. He'd hated the role he'd played in separating them from their daughter, even if it was unconsciously done.

"But how are *you* feeling about it?" His mom clucked her tongue at him. "I know they're happy to see her. But she isn't my concern. You are. And I'm worried about what seeing her is gonna do to you."

He opened his mouth to tell her that the idea of seeing Jessie again hurt, but then it dawned on him that it really didn't. He closed his mouth without speaking as he rolled that realization around in his head. The knowledge that he was going to see the woman who left him standing at the altar actually didn't hurt.

Had he really and truly moved on, then?

"Dexter?" His mom put a hand on his shoulder and he looked up. Her eyes were clouded with concern. "I knew I should have found a way to keep them from inviting her. This is too much for you."

"No. It's fine. Really." The way to explain it finally came to him. "I realized just now that it no longer bothered me that I might have to see Jessie again. I know... I know... I've been saying for a while that I was over her. But I don't think I was. At least not fully."

"And you are now?"

He hadn't known hope could be audible until that moment, but he heard the hope in his mother's voice as she asked that.

"I am," he confirmed, flashing her a real smile. "I really am."

"Lena is more than just good for you, then," his mom said, her voice no longer concerned but now filled with a happiness he hadn't heard directed at him in years. "I think I'm going to love that girl."

He was going to have to burst that happiness bubble like a bully would pop a younger child's balloon when he told her that he and Lena "broke up" after the holidays. And he stubbornly shoved away the thought that maybe, just maybe, Lena's presence in his life was why he finally felt completely over Jessie. Accepting that would make things with Lena far too real.

Lena paused outside the doorway to the kitchen as she overheard the tail end of Dex's conversation with his mother about his ex. Hearing him say that he was completely over Jessie sent a warmth running through her entire body that made her giddy. She wanted to find some pompoms and do a cheer. Or clap like a lunatic until she burst into awkward laughter.

She wasn't ready to acknowledge why Dex's confession made her so happy she could skip. But it really and truly did.

Taking several deep breaths, she tried to wipe the smile from her lips that would clue him in that she'd overheard his conversation.

Making sure to make her steps heavy, she took the final few steps into the kitchen. She poured herself a cup of coffee and walked over to him. She couldn't stop herself from wrapping her arms around his waist and giving him a tight hug from behind.

"So, uh, what's the plan for today?" she

tried to ask nonchalantly. Like she hadn't been eavesdropping on their conversation from the hallway. "I know the rehearsal dinner is tomorrow, but is there anything on the schedule today?"

"We are having lunch with the soon-to-be newlyweds and her parents," Dex's mom said. A pained look crossed her face and she added, "And some family from each side."

"What my mama is hinting at, unsuccessfully, is that Jessie is likely to be there."

"I see…" Lena leaned against Dex, trying to work out how she was supposed to feel at the thought of meeting the ex before the wedding. "Do I have anything to worry about with her?"

"Of course not," Dex protested, stiffening up beneath her touch.

"Then bring it on. I'm looking forward to meeting the rest of your family, at least. I thought there'd be more people here this morning, even."

Namely, Dex's father and the aunt from the next room they'd had to be quiet for to avoid waking. When she'd come downstairs in search of food and coffee this morning, she'd found only Mrs. Henry sitting and staring out over the most beautiful sunrise Lena had ever seen.

"David and Peggy went into Gatlinburg for

the morning. Every time Peggy is here, she insists on having a morning with just the two of them, and they usually end up at the Donut Friar to get her cinnamon bread fix in."

Dex laughed. "But it's so good that I can't even blame her for that. Lena, I'll take you if we have time before we leave."

Seeing his comment as the perfect way to reinforce his mom's belief in their fake relationship, Lena laid her head on Dex's shoulder. "If not this time, maybe we can do it next time, then."

His mom had been kind this morning, but she'd gotten the impression that the older woman wasn't completely buying that they were in love. Not even after walking in on them kissing last night. She was very perceptive and had a way of looking at a person that made them want to spill every secret they'd ever heard.

They'd have to up their game to make it through this week without being found out. But Lena was up for the challenge. She'd handled twenty-seven years under her parents' scrutiny. One week under the watchful eye of the Henry matriarch would be a breeze.

Meeting the ex was what she was more worried about. This Jessie had dated and loved Dex for years, so she'd know his tells and mannerisms. If anyone was going to out them as fake, it would be her.

"Where are we meeting everyone for lunch?" Dex asked.

"Down at Westfield Steak House. Roy and Mary reserved their party room. And tomorrow morning we will head over to the church and get all the decorations up before having the rehearsal and that awful ugly sweater party that Jill insists on."

Dex and his mom talked about some of the people who might be there, with Mrs. Henry filling Dex in on what had happened with them regularly.

The mention of Jill's parents brought questions to mind for Lena. Even if they managed to pull the fake relationship off for the entire week here, Dex would have to deal with his ex being around for the rest of his life with his brother marrying her sister. What would he do next time? Find another fake girlfriend? She mentally noted to bring this up with him when they were alone.

Wade stumbled into the kitchen just then, half-asleep and half-dressed. "I'm hungry."

Mrs. Henry looked him up and down without a word.

Lena knew there was something being said with the older woman's gaze, she just wasn't sure what. Wade must have understood though, because he left and returned a minute later fully dressed.

When he sat next to Dex, a plate of pancakes was placed in front of him. He tucked in like he'd never eaten before. Like Dex, his appetite surprised Lena.

"Wow, I can't imagine what your grocery bill was like when all of your boys were at home."

Mrs. Henry laughed. "More than a mortgage payment for years. Are you hungry? I think that batter you made is salvageable. I can make you up some pancakes if you don't think you can wait for lunch."

"No, but thank you." Lena shook her head. If she ate even a third of what she'd seen Dex put away, she'd be sick. "I'm good to wait."

"Lena…" Wade said with a grin. "You look more beautiful in the light of day. You know, you could move across the hall and get to know the better Henry man."

Dex slugged him in the arm. "Hey! Back off."

Lena couldn't help but laugh. "I'm afraid I

can't take you up on that, but it was, uh, sweet of you to offer."

"Sweet? You think he's sweet?" Dex shot her a look of pure disbelief. "There ain't nothing sweet about Wade."

"Is this why you wanted to give him away?"

"Give me away!" Wade gasped in faked outrage. "How dare you? Dex, I'm hurt."

"Lena's never had a sibling." Dex shrugged nonchalantly, but the look he shot his brother was one hundred percent mischief. "I told her I had a spare."

"Well, Dexter, I'm not sure which is worse, giving Wade to Lena because she was an only child or selling Tommy for a potato."

Lena nearly spit out her coffee. "You sold him for a potato?"

The slightest hint of a blush crept up into Dex's cheeks, but he met her gaze defiantly. His eyes crinkled up in that happy way she loved. "In my defense, that potato was shaped like a duck. Wade's proof that a kid can have another baby brother, but how often do you find a potato that looks like a duck?"

"You need a little more backstory before you judge my son too hard on this. He was only two, after all. And Tommy had the worst colic. That child…he didn't sleep for more than a few minutes at a time and I usually had to be walking the floors with him to get him to doze off then."

"That sounds rough."

"Dexter had been so excited to get a baby brother." A soft smile lit her face as she reminisced about Dex as a child, and Lena could see hints of Dex in the crinkles around her eyes. "I think Tommy was a bit of a disappointment since all he did was cry and puke. My daddy had just retired and had a big garden that year. He used that garden to keep Dexter busy for me so that I could focus on Tommy. When Dexter dug up that duck potato, he wanted to keep it. Well, Daddy told him he had to pay for it if he wanted to keep it."

"To be fair, my first offer was my fire truck. But then I tripped and broke the duck potato." Dex stretched, his shirt pulling tight across his muscular chest. "And I couldn't trade a perfectly good fire truck for a broken potato. So I offered him a broken baby brother."

"Wow."

"Yeah, as you can see, it's been three whole decades and I still haven't lived that one down. I'll be hearing about it until I'm old and gray." Dex grinned at her and she could tell he wasn't upset in the slightest by his family's teasing.

In fact, she thought he might like it.

There was a warmth in this room that had nothing to do with the heating and entirely to do with the love shared by the people in it. It seeped in through the soft smiles and was reinforced with the patted shoulders. It was something Lena had absolutely no experience with.

She'd never had her mother look at her with the kind of indulgent tenderness that Mrs. Henry did her sons. Her mother had never made her a single meal and certainly wouldn't have gotten up early just to have a moment alone before doing it.

What would it have been like to have been surrounded by pure affection her entire life?

A longing rose up in her chest. She wanted what Dex had with his family. The fondness and caring, even the teasing, made her yearn for the impossible.

Sitting in that kitchen, surrounded by Dex and his family, in that instant, it felt very possible. If Dex ever attempted something long-term again, that is.

But even more, would she ever be able to live up to the expectations of a family like this? She had no experience with what a healthy, loving relationship looked like. Romantic or platonic.

A shrill song pierced the moment and Lena

blinked several times while she tried to focus on where the sound was coming from. Finally, she dug her cell phone out of her pocket and winced as the caller's name flashed on the screen.

Of course. The woman had a sixth sense for knowing when happiness crossed Lena's path and her instinct was to burst that bubble. Fast.

Lena put the phone to her ear. "Hello, Mother."

# CHAPTER ELEVEN

LENA SCHOOLED HER expression to a calm facade, but Dex had spent enough time with her to catch the frustration and hint of fear. Talking to her mother scared her?

For a split second, he wanted to jump up and pull her into his arms, reassure her that she wasn't going to have to face her parents alone. Then common sense returned and the recollection that this was entirely a farce washed over him with a grim reality.

He wouldn't be there beyond this single visit. And he couldn't let himself forget that simple fact.

She met his gaze and then motioned toward the door. At his nod, she stepped out onto the back deck to take her call. Through the windows, he watched her pace, tension in her frame visible through the glass.

"She doesn't get on well with her mama,

does she?" Wade asked around a bite of pancakes.

"That's an understatement." It wasn't his place to share all of Lena's secrets, but the answer to Wade's question was pretty obvious. "So, what's going on today in Westfield?"

Changing the subject to the town's Christmas traditions was as much a tactic to distract himself as Wade. He didn't want to accidentally share something Lena might have told him in confidence.

"Oh, you're in luck. They are having a gingerbread house contest over at the library at four, and I believe the Mason lodge has a craft fair going on." His mom pursed her lips in thought. "At least, I think they do. You'll have to drive by the lodge and see. I might have the dates mixed up on that one."

"I thought I'd take Lena out and spend some one-on-one time doing something Christmassy after lunch. I already have tickets for the High Bridge in Gatlinburg. I want to show her the lights later tonight."

"Just the two of you?" Wade whistled low and slow. "That sounds romantic. You aren't about to pop the question too, are you? I'm not even ready to be the only Henry man left single."

*Propose?*

Oh, man. He hadn't thought out the implications of taking her to the High Bridge alone at night. While he knew Lena would not be expecting a proposal that evening, he hadn't considered how it would look to his family for him to take her to one of the most romantic spots in the area. He glanced over at his mom and she'd perked up at the conversation. Her eyes were lit with excitement that he had to crush.

"Uh, no. I was just thinking that since she loves Christmas so much, she'd like to see the lights over Gatlinburg and the mountains. We haven't been dating that long and we aren't at that point yet."

"You said you saw a future with her, though?" his mom questioned. "Why wouldn't you propose?"

"Yeah," he said, gesturing vaguely. He swallowed hard. Fake dating was one thing, but he refused to propose. That was too far. "In the future. Don't rush it, Mama. I've known her less than a year."

"I knew your father was the man for me after our first date." His mom smiled at him knowingly. "He proposed on our third date. By the time we'd known each other a year, we were married and expecting you."

"If you follow their timeline, I'll be an uncle by next Christmas." Wade grinned at him, mischief filling his face. "'Uncle Wade' has a nice ring to it."

"Hush."

"Seriously, though, if you don't mind taking her someplace with a lot of, uh, old memories, the ice rink has open skate this afternoon."

Dex snorted. "If I only took her to places in Westfield where I'd never taken Jessie, I could only take her to places built after the breakup. It's a small town. Jessie and I went everywhere here, especially if it was even slightly romantic."

As high school sweethearts, he and Jessie had probably found every niche and alcove in the town where they could share a few kisses and fumbled fondles. They'd had more than a few dates at the ice rink in town, but it held no special significance to him. No major firsts had occurred there, unlike the little theater down by the courthouse, where he'd had his first ever kiss, or the church they'd be standing in for Tommy and Jill's wedding, where she'd left him at the altar. He couldn't avoid memories of Jessie in Westfield. He could only make new ones here with Lena.

"Maybe I'll just see what Lena wants to do

today. Give her the options and let her choose."
He pushed back from the counter. Standing, he
put his plate and coffee mug in the dishwasher.
"Thanks for breakfast, Mama. I'm going to
take Lena's coat out to her before she freezes
out there."

Grabbing her jacket—and one of his brother's jackets for himself since his own was covered with blood—he stepped out on the deck
and caught a snippet of Lena's conversation.

"Yes, Dex will be attending with me. I did
RSVP for myself and a plus one for a reason."

She smiled up at him softly when he wrapped
her coat around her shivering shoulders. She
mouthed a *thank you* at him before rolling her
eyes at something her mother must have said.

"I know that, Mother. And believe me, I
am fully aware of the expectations that you
and Father have for my behavior. I trust Dexter to behave in an appropriate manner." Her
lips thinned out to a barely visible line. She
grew silent and while he couldn't make out the
words, he could just make out that her mother
was lecturing on the other end of the call.

The seriousness on her face and the formal
way she spoke to her mother struck him as unacceptable. Today was supposed to be a fun day
and he didn't want to let her mother ruin that

for her. The witch had already stolen the sparkle from Lena's eyes. Needing to see her smile, Dex stuck his thumbs to his ears and wiggled his fingers while making a cross-eyed face.

Lena snorted and spun away from him. "Of course I wasn't laughing at you. That was a sneeze."

She looked back over at him and grinned. Her shoulders shook in silent laughter, and her eyes once again contained a glint of delight.

*Mission accomplished.*

"I'm sorry, Mother, but I really do need to go. We are attending a luncheon with his parents and it would be unacceptable for me to be late."

She ended the call and stepped up to him, pressing her face against his chest. His heart thudded against his rib cage as she wrapped her arms around his waist.

"Thank you for that," she murmured, her voice muffled. "She drives me crazy."

"I could tell."

"Lecturing me about behaving in a manner befitting a Franklin while I'm here as well as at the gala, as if I hadn't attended dozens of formal events at their sides throughout the years. I think if I'd told her you were standing next to me, she'd have given you a lecture on expectations as well. Actually, you should probably expect one once we get to California."

The loud sigh of resignation Lena gave sank deep.

"Well, if she gives me a lecture, I promise not to hold it against you. We really do need to head out soon to get to the restaurant on time, but you have time to change if you want."

"Is my outfit unacceptable?" Lena stiffened against him.

*Open mouth, insert foot.*

"You look amazing. I did *not* mean to imply otherwise. I have this condition where my mouth works faster than my brain. It gets me in trouble a lot." Squeezing her close, he pressed a kiss to the top of her head. "After lunch, what do you say to a craft fair or ice skating?"

"Changing the subject from your gaffe?"

"Trying to." He tipped her head up to his and met her eyes. "You really do look stunning. This isn't going to be anything formal, so jeans and a sweater are perfect."

"Mmm-hmm."

"So, will you spend the afternoon with me?"

"Are you asking me on another fake date?" Mischief brightened her expression.

"Who said it was fake?"

The pull to put his lips to hers nearly got

the best of him. He'd been aching to kiss her since he walked into the kitchen to find her with flour on her face. When her arms slid up around his neck and she rose up on tiptoe, he groaned. Tightening his arms around her, he pressed his forehead to hers. His voice was low and ragged when he said, "We kiss and this is real."

Lena stiffened. She dropped down from her toes and moved to step back. "Didn't you say we had somewhere to be?"

"Hmm... I think the lunch is optional." He tried to bring her back into his embrace, but she was too evasive.

"Nice try." Lena stepped away from him, and this time he allowed the separation. "I'm pretty sure that as the best man, your presence is expected."

"But I get some alone time later, right?" he negotiated, knowing she was right. He had to attend. Not attending would get him strung up by his ears. But in this moment, he wanted to convince Lena to take a risk on him. Only then could he get her out of his system. "An actual real date?"

Smiling at him a little shyly, Lena nodded. Her voice was soft when she said, "I think I'd like that."

\* \* \*

A short while later, Dex ushered her to his SUV so they could head into town. Butterflies fluttered about in her stomach and she couldn't decide if it was in remembrance of the embraces on the Henry's back deck or worries about meeting his ex-fiancée.

Westfield was a twisty maze of narrow streets that flowed along the side of the mountain. And the curves did nothing to settle her stomach.

"Are you sure we have to do this?" Dex slowed to a stop to allow a group of kids to run across a brick crosswalk to the playground on the opposite side. "It's not too late to make a break for it and head back to Nashville."

"Ha!" Lena poked playfully at Dex's arm. "Only if you tell your mother face-to-face, because I don't want the fallout of her finding out after the fact that you snuck out of town like the paparazzi are hiding behind every bush."

Groaning, Dex turned right. "This is going to be horrendous."

"I hate to see what you'll think of my family dinners, then. Your family is nothing compared to mine. Trust me. We got this."

She tamped down her nerves. Promises had been made and she wouldn't go back on them.

Turning her gaze to the view outside the car window, Lena focused on the uniqueness of the little town. City planning seemed lax and every building appeared to have been borrowed from a different architectural era. Somehow, it fit together as a beautiful and cohesive patchwork.

Dex pulled to a stop in front of the steakhouse. "Not sure I'm ready for this."

"Seeing her again?" Lena asked, placing her hand over his.

"Yeah." He winced. "Sorry, I guess I shouldn't have said that since I have you here as my date. I didn't mean..."

"I know you didn't mean anything by it. I'm not sure I'll ever be ready to see Connor again." She sighed. A century would be too soon, but there was a good chance he'd be at the New Year's Eve gala, and that thought was sobering.

Taking her hand in his, Dex brought it up to his lips and pressed a soft kiss on her wrist. "He didn't deserve you."

"I know."

Dex laughed. "Good to see you found a little of your self-esteem, at least."

At barely more than a whisper, she confessed, "It's only because I'm with you. You make me feel like I'm really worth something."

"Good." His gaze was hot and intense. "I really want to kiss you right now."

She cupped his cheek with her palm. "I'm not stopping you."

With a groan, Dex leaned across the center console to kiss her but stopped a breath away from their lips meeting when there was a tap on the glass. He muttered a curse under his breath before straightening up.

An older version of Dex stood outside the vehicle, grinning from ear to ear.

"My dad," Dex explained unnecessarily. He turned the SUV off and got out, hugging his dad and laughing.

*Why can't I have that?*

Again, Lena found herself envious of his relationship with his parents. Her dad would never hug her like that in public. He barely offered the occasional hug in private. They just didn't have a lovey-dovey relationship.

When—if—she ever had children, she'd make sure they knew they were loved and wanted from the moment of conception, and not merely because she wanted an heir. She wanted them to have the same carefree joy that Dex must have had in childhood to have such a warm personality and loving relationship with his family. The more she got to know him, the more she saw the truth of the man inside. And the more she liked. Oh, boy, did she like what she saw when she looked at Dex.

Sighing, she reached for the door handle just to have the door opened before she could touch it. Another Henry male stood in the opening. Same dark hair, same broad frame, but this one had a beard darkening his jawline.

"I'm guessing you are Tommy," she said.

Grinning down at her, he nodded. "And you must be Lena. I've heard so much about you."

She glanced toward Dex. "Oh?"

"You've really gotten to him, you know. And from that smile on his face, I'd say that's a very good thing." Tommy held a hand out and assisted her out of the vehicle. "It's good to see him happy again."

Smiling back at Tommy, she said, "He makes me happy too."

The thoughts of her and Dex making each other happy flooded her mind and sparked a boatload of questions. Was Dex a good actor? Or was he really and truly happier than he had been the last time his family had seen him? And if he was happier, then what part did she play?

Before the landslide of emotions tied to those questions took her out, Lena let a tease slip from her lips uncensored. "Did the sale fall through once the potato was gone or did your grandfather return you as defective merchandise?"

"Ha!" Tommy chuckled, loud and deep. His laugh had a similar sound to Dex's but it didn't affect her like his brother's did. "They told you about that, huh?"

She eyed him up and down. "I'd have sold you for a snow cone."

Tommy laughed harder. His eyes watered and he was gasping for air before he could get his breathing under control. "I bet you don't take any sass, do you? You couldn't be more perfect for Dex if you tried."

Tommy's words warmed her heart. She smiled over at Dex, who was still on the other side of the SUV talking to his dad, and he winked when they made eye contact.

She loved the way he seemed aware of her, even when he wasn't right at her side. It made her feel loved, more than she'd ever had with Connor or anyone else she'd dated.

*Oh, no.*

Closing her eyes, she swallowed hard. She couldn't start loving things about Dex! That wasn't part of the plan. This was spiraling out of her control. And she'd already agreed to go on a real date with him later today. Nervous energy washed over her. What had she gotten herself into?

"Hey, you okay?" Dex asked, putting a hand on her shoulder. "You just got really pale all of a sudden."

With a forced smile, she nodded. "I just need to eat, I think."

Wrapping his arm around her waist, he leaned in close. Whispering softly in her ear, he asked, "Are you sure that's all? You could tell me if there was something bothering you. I'll find a way to fix it."

He'd come around the vehicle in seconds once he'd noticed her reaction. How could she not fall for a man who cared enough to watch her expressions like Dex did? He was so observant. Now more than ever, Lena couldn't believe any woman would be stupid enough to leave him standing at the altar.

She leaned her head against Dex's chest and inhaled his scent. "I'm okay. Really."

But was she?

She was falling in love with Dexter Henry, playboy general surgeon. Despite the warnings and initial red flags, Dex was a genuinely good man. That's what made him so easy to fall for. He was kind, considerate, and had a smile that could unlock the most guarded of hearts. But Dex had made it crystal clear that he was only looking for short-term. She had no doubts he'd be interested in kicking their fake relationship up to a full-blown sexual relationship for the duration of the holidays, but it was the concern about what happened when they went back to Nashville in January that gave her pause.

If they got involved and then he stuck to his love 'em and leave 'em pattern, she'd have to look at him every single day at work. She'd gone that route with Connor and the fallout had sent her fleeing across the country when the full details of their unfortunate affair reached the lips of the rumor mill. Where would she go if things with Dex blew up at Metro Memorial?

She sighed and snuggled in closer to his chest. Which was the exact opposite of what she should be doing... She took a deep breath and his scent filled her nostrils. This would be so much easier if Dex didn't feel and smell like home.

He whispered in her ear, "Are you ready to do this? I'm not sure I am, but I feel like I can face her finally with you at my side. You give me strength."

Heart slamming into her ribs, Lena tried not to read too much into his words. Really, she did. But his words gave her hope that he was starting to think long-term, and maybe, just maybe, falling for her like she was falling for him. Hope led to excitement. If he was feeling the same, maybe they could make this more than a holiday fling.

Filling her lungs with Dex-scented air, Lena straightened her spine and pulled her courage around her like a protective cloak. Her mother and her grandparents before her were pillars of Los Angeles society, and Lena could fake her way through an awkward dinner with the best of them.

"Absolutely," she said, pleased to hear that there was not even a hint of a quiver in her voice. "Let's get this meeting over with and get some food. I'm hungry."

# CHAPTER TWELVE

DEX LED LENA inside the restaurant, guiding her with his hand on the small of her back. He wasn't sure what had upset her outside, but something had. She seemed to have put it out of her mind, though. She had a smile on her face and held her head high as she walked by his side. Still, something about the way her eyes shifted around the restaurant was less curiosity at new surroundings and more nervousness.

Tommy motioned them toward the back room where the party was being held. He hadn't stopped smiling today. Tommy had found his perfect match and Dex had never been happier for him.

He steeled his resolve as they stepped through the doorway into the reserved room. His mom sat at the end of the table just inside the door talking to Mary. Mary had a cell phone in her hand, swiping through what looked like a series of beach pictures. His future sister-in-law, Jill, was at the far end of the room. The smile on Jill's face was as big as the one on his brother's as she stood there talking to his aunt Peggy. He recognized one of Jill and Jessie's aunts sitting with Ray.

But the one person he'd expected to see wasn't there.

He looked around, thinking somehow he'd missed her, but no. Jessie wasn't there. A wave of frustration washed over him. He'd been ready to see her, ready to get this first meeting over with, and it was a letdown to find that she wasn't there.

"Dexter!" Ray saw him and came over. The older man started to give him a hug, but then switched it at the last second to an awkward handshake. "It's been a long time. How have you been?"

Years ago, Ray would have hugged him, no question. Now, though? It was awkward. The pain of that resonated deep in his gut. He and Ray had always had a good relationship. Jessie had broken that too.

Okay, maybe he'd contributed by vanishing to Nashville and barely returning, but Ray hadn't reached out to him, either.

"I'm good, Ray." He took Lena's hand in his.

"I'd like you to meet my girlfriend, Lena." He made the introductions and some small talk with Ray for a few minutes. He wanted to ask where Jessie was, but he didn't out of respect for the woman at his side.

Ray began to look uncomfortable. He shifted from one foot to the other and didn't make eye contact when he asked, "Uh, Dex, you did hear that Jessie's coming home for the wedding, right?"

Just the opening he needed.

"I did, actually. I'm glad to hear it. I can only imagine how much you and Mary have been missing her. You haven't seen her since our rehearsal dinner, have you?" He rubbed his thumb along Lena's hand, hoping to keep her aware that he was grateful for her presence.

"Not once. She didn't even call us for the first year or so." Ray sighed, rubbing the bridge of his nose. "But she's promised Jill and Mary that she'd be here for this wedding."

He didn't look happy about that fact. And Dex didn't blame him. They'd always been such a close family. It had to be eating at them that she'd abandoned her family like that.

"Ah, well, then the wedding's serving a dual purpose?"

With a wry smile, Ray shrugged. "I'll believe she's coming in when I see her. She called and said they bumped her flight back until tomorrow night. She's still supposed to be here in time for the wedding, though."

So he had another day without having to face her. He could live with that. "At least you'll have her home for Christmas this year."

"True, true." Ray smiled at Lena. "I hope we aren't upsetting you with our conversation about Jessie. I'm sure she's the last thing you'd choose for a topic."

Lena handled his concerns with aplomb. "No worries at all. Dex told me about his relationship with your daughter. It's only natural that you'd speak of the connection. Now, it's your youngest daughter that's marrying his brother, is that right?"

The smoothness of Lena's transition from Jessie and the past to Jill and the present made Dex smile. Ray seemed impressed as well. How could he not be? Lena was poised and confident, not to mention beautiful.

Her composure held as he introduced her to the rest of his family. She kept that smile on her face even when stories were told of his past with Jessie. When they had a moment of relative privacy, he questioned her about it.

"I can't believe it doesn't bother you at all

when they bring up my past. I know if your family starts telling stories of you and your ex, I'm going to be a jealous mess. What's your secret?"

She leaned close and her lips brushed his earlobe as she answered. "We have her to thank for our chance at being together. If she hadn't crushed you, you'd have never needed me to come home with you. So thank her, don't hate her."

*Thank her, don't hate her.*

Those five words changed everything for him. He looked at Lena, and it dawned on him that his future really was sitting next to him in a soft blue sweater. Not just a short fling, but a real future. And the thought scared him senseless.

He wasn't looking for forever. He wanted fun and easy and low risk. But if that was true, then why was Lena tempting him to throw all those wants to the side and risk it all?

Lena made him feel more alive than he'd felt in years. The protective walls he'd erected around his heart were being cracked open, and the desire to knock them down entirely so that he could give Lena his whole heart was getting hard to resist.

Mary and his mom called for everyone to

sit. All the tables had been pushed into one huge table that took up most of the vast space. Dark cloths covered the table, and several bright flower arrangements were placed at evenly spaced intervals along the table. Servers started bringing in food, family style.

He found himself seated between his dad and Lena, who seemed to hit it off instantly. At one point, he just reclined back to make it easier for them to continue their discussion. Usually his dad's financial discussions ended up a little over his head, but Lena had a surprising knowledge of finances. From the gleam in his dad's eyes, Lena had won him over in that single conversation.

Watching her banter back and forth with Wade brought a smile to Dex's face. She was holding her own against his annoying little brother, and even more, she seemed to be enjoying it.

Seeing her fit in with his family felt so strange. He'd convinced himself that Lena was such a city girl that his family would make short work of her and he could use that as justification for why they "broke up" in a few weeks. Somehow, he'd really thought this week would be easy justification for why their relationship ended. Yet Lena was not only getting along easily, but she was even bonding with them.

He wanted to have her bond with him. He rubbed the bridge of his nose. Jealous of his own family? That was a new low for him. And maybe a hint of warning that he was getting in over his head with Lena. But rather than reinforcing the walls around his heart, he reached for her hand and their fingers interlocked. She smiled softly over at him before returning to her conversation with his dad and brother.

Shortly after they'd finished eating, he leaned over and asked her quietly, "You wanna get out of here? How's ice skating sound?"

She nodded.

Within five minutes, they were back in his SUV and heading down to the local ice rink.

"I haven't been ice skating since I was a teenager," she said with a laugh. "And not even regularly then. I'm not sure I'm going to be any good at this, but I'm game to try it."

He wanted to pull her close and hoped that skating would give him the opportunity. "All you have to do is hold my hand, and I promise, I'll never let you fall."

"On the ice or in life?" she asked.

He wasn't sure he had the words to communicate everything he was feeling. Slipping his hand over hers, he squeezed gently. "I want to be with you, Lena. I want to see where this could go between us."

"For how long, though?" She pulled her hand away and tucked it into her coat pocket.

While he wasn't completely sure, he thought she was saying she wanted something long-term. He knew she'd hated how he bounced from relationship to relationship, and she'd said she didn't want this to be real. But occasionally she said something that made him think she'd be open to more if there was the possibility of a commitment.

Even a day ago, he'd have sworn he wasn't the commitment type anymore.

But how long did it take for a woman to change a man's mind?

A month? A week?

The breadth of a kiss?

Lena's muscles tensed as Dex pulled her around the ice rink. She clung to his hands like he was her lifeline, her only defense against another bone-jarring crash into the ice at their feet. Her savior—he'd rescued her from a few hard falls. His protective nature and gentle coaxing as he'd tried to teach her to ice-skate had given her a glimpse at the type of father

Dex would be, if he could ever open his heart up to a long-term relationship again.

"I think you are starting to get the hang of this," Dex encouraged as he skated backward, holding both of Lena's hands in his own. He glided across the ice with a grace she envied.

"Ha, you're only saying that because the last time I fell I didn't take you out with me." Unlike the time before where she'd slammed him into the wall so hard that a hockey ref would have called a penalty on her for boarding. She'd managed to knock the breath out of them both in one embarrassing moment.

"That might bear a slight resemblance to the truth." He laughed. The chill of the ice rink had added color to his cheeks. "Are you having fun, at least?"

"I'm freezing cold and have bruised far more than my pride, but surprisingly, yes, I am having fun." Her right skate hit a divot in the ice and she pitched forward into his chest. "But I swear this skate has it out for me."

Thankfully, he had enough balance for the both of them and kept them from tumbling onto the ice again. His arms wrapped around her, keeping her upright. "I'm sure it's the skate's fault. You want me to give it a good talking to?"

"If you think it will help," she murmured from her position against his chest. "I think I'll sit this lap out and maybe get some hot chocolate. Not sure my bottom can handle another hard landing."

A group of teenagers skated past, laughing. Cheeks pink from the cold, they seemed far surer on those tiny strips of metal strapped to their feet than Lena could ever hope to be. She watched one of the girls do some fancy loop or axel—Lena wasn't sure of the proper terminology. Even a child had more technical ability on the ice than she did.

"She's good," Dex said.

Lena looked up at him in question. How'd he know what she'd been thinking?

"You've been watching her. If she's who I think she is, her grandparents own this rink, so she's practically grown up here." He brushed Lena's hair back and tucked it behind her ear. "She's been skating as long as she could walk, so of course she's good."

"So, what you are saying is that I shouldn't feel bad that someone who is half my age is a better skater than me?"

He whispered in her ear, "I'm sure there are a lot of things that you are far better at than that kid is."

She blushed at his comment, feeling the heat rising up into her cheeks at the innuendo in his words. "Shh…what if the kids hear?"

He shrugged. "So what if they do? You are a great nurse. None of them would be of any help at all in surgery. Most of them probably barely know basic anatomy."

Pushing against his chest, she moved away from him, wobbling on her skates. "That's not what you meant."

"If anyone overheard me, it is exactly what I meant." The broad smile on his face was as innocent as it was genuine. "I'll defend that position to the end too."

Lena grabbed for the rail when her skate decided to go off on its own again. "How 'bout that hot chocolate?"

Answering physically rather than verbally, Dex led her off the ice and over to the food counter. He ordered them a couple hot chocolates, and they went and sat on one of the benches overlooking the rink. It was a little warmer off the ice, at least.

"I'm so cold I think my blood has frozen." Cupping her hands around the warm cup of chocolate, Lena sighed. "And don't even lecture me on how that's impossible. I may not have a medical degree, but I know how I feel. And that's nearly solid ice."

He wrapped an arm around her shoulders and leaned in close. His breath was warm and delicious against her cheek. "If you didn't insist on sitting on the ice so much, you wouldn't be chilled through."

"We don't have winter where I'm from!" she protested. "Even the coldest days are warmer than it is in here. How'd you do the last time you went surfing?"

A loud, harsh laugh burst out of him and drew the attention of some of the people around them. "I've never attempted to surf, so probably worse than you did skating. Do you surf?"

"I used to." There was a longing in her voice. Man, she missed the rush of being out on the waves. The freedom that came with being out on the water. But when Dex picked up her hand and held it in his own, she missed it a little bit less.

"Well, I know just the thing to cheer you up. It's not surfing, but I'm sure you going to love it anyway." He squeezed her close and pressed a kiss to her temple. "Way better than ice skating, I promise."

Her heart raced at that tiny display of intimacy. "What do you have planned?"

"If I tell, it ruins the surprise." He stood and offered her his hand. "Do you trust me?"

She gazed up at him while she considered the question. Did she trust him? He had such an earnest expression on his face in that moment that not taking his hand had to be a crime. Gingerly, she placed her hand in his.

"I'm going to trust you for the evening."

A wide grin spread across his face. "You won't regret it."

Leading her out of the skating rink, he had her tucked into the passenger seat of the SUV before either of them uttered another word. When he turned the SUV out of town and back down the twisty road they'd traveled when they came in from Gatlinburg, she had to speak up.

"Where exactly are you taking me?" She gasped as they passed several white-tailed deer standing right on the side of the road. "Did you see them?"

"Everyday occurrence around here." He glanced over at her. "You look shocked. Have you never seen deer before?"

Lena scoffed. "Not outside a zoo or nature preserve. City girl, remember? We don't exactly have deer running past the hospital in LA. I mean, in some of the parks and on the outskirts, yeah, but not where I'm from."

"Don't look to the left now if deer shock you."

"A bear!" She spun in her seat and her excited exclamation filled the cab. Staring out the window, Lena could barely believe her eyes as Dex drove slowly past the large black bear who seemed to be in no hurry as she lumbered down the road. "Don't bears hibernate? Why is it just ambling down the road right now instead of sleeping?"

"Ah, see, that's what most people think. But where it stays warmer here, our bears don't spend months straight hibernating like northern bears do. They do sleep for extended periods, of course. But they are also very easily awakened. And when they wake up they usually go searching for food and stay up for a little while before they return to their den or sometimes find a new one."

"I had no idea." She tried to sneak a topic change in while he was in a talkative mood. "So, where are you taking me for our first real date? It's getting dark now."

"We are almost there." He reached over and squeezed her hand briefly. "Did skating not count as a real date? By my count, this should be date number two."

"Nice try. Same day, same date."

His mention of this being a real date sent her heart out for a jog. Dating for real made her nervous, and excited, and a thousand other emotions all at once. Lena's mind raced as they passed by tourist attraction after tourist attraction. "Are we doing a dinner theater show?"

"Nope."

"Can I get a little hint?" Christmas lights competed with attraction signs in every direction. Twinkling lights lit all the trees along the sidewalks, and most of the businesses had lighted displays garnishing their windows, filled with Santas and reindeer-pulled sleighs.

"Nope."

"Are we buying moonshine?" She laughed as they drove past a second distillery. "I never had moonshine but I'm not opposed to trying it."

"That's not why we are here, but we can stop in to one of the distilleries on the way back if you like."

"Hmm…" She scanned the signs along the street. "I don't think it's the aquarium."

"Nope." He pulled into a public parking lot. "We have to walk a bit to get where we are going."

Interest piqued, Lena climbed out of the

SUV and wrapped her scarf tighter against the cold wind. "Is it indoors?"

Dex gave an awkward sounding chuckle. "Not exactly, but give it a chance, okay?"

They walked a block or so down, with Lena completely fascinated by the red lifts going up the side of the mountain into the darkness. Above them, a suspension bridge hung, covered in Christmas lights.

"Are we going up there?" she asked, her voice as filled with wonder as a small child's on Christmas morning.

"Yeah, we are. I hope you aren't afraid of heights."

He showed their tickets to the attendant and they were soon seated in the next lift chair. The attendant tucked the safety bar down into place and they began the slow trek up the mountain.

"This is amazing, but cold!"

Dex's arm settled over her shoulders and the weight brought with it a delicious warmth much welcome in the crisp evening air. "Does this help? If not, I can think of a few other ways to warm you up."

The words sounded like a flirtatious challenge as they rolled off his tongue, but Lena didn't want to run away from something with Dex anymore. Being with Dex, spending time with him and seeing how he was when with his family, had changed her opinions on giving a relationship a chance.

She loved him. Loved spending time with him.

*Love...*

She swallowed back the realization that she'd somehow allowed herself to fall in love with Dex. No longer falling, she was head over heels, beyond the point of rescue. She laid her head on his shoulder. What would come next? How on earth did she proceed with a fake relationship when she was in real love with the surgeon at her side?

When they reached the top and got off the lift, employees ushered them inside to warm up. Dex bought them each a hot chocolate, and they sat up on the second floor, staring out over the town below them.

"This place is gorgeous." Wisps of steam rose from the mug in her hands and warmed her wind-chilled cheeks. "I'd love to see the fall color from up here."

"Maybe next fall. My mom would love to show you all the touristy places around Westfield too. It's kinda her thing, after all." Dex sipped at his own drink. "But there's one more part to this evening and I think it will be your favorite."

Confidence abounded in his voice. The wind had put color in his face. Women from across the room eyed him and not even discreetly. In jeans today, or scrubs at the hospital, Dex was a man who drew attention with very little effort. It felt really good to have his attention focused on her.

When she finished her hot chocolate, Dex took her hand.

"Come on, one last thing before we head back down the mountain." He led her outside and over to the suspension bridge she'd been in awe of from down in town. "You ready for this?"

The suspension bridge seemed to extend forever. Christmas lights lit up the railings and some of the cables all the way across the valley, it seemed. Bright reds, greens and blues twinkled in rows above their heads and at their sides. As they stepped out onto the bridge, Lena gaped at the glass panels at their feet and the rows of lights below them too.

"Dex, this is…wow."

When they reached the center of the bridge, Dex stopped her. "I thought you might like to see Gatlinburg lit up for Christmas from the best view in town."

"It's beautiful."

His arm slipped around her waist and moved her into his embrace. Tilting her chin up, he leaned in close. "So are you."

Lena couldn't fight the attraction anymore. When her arms snaked up around his neck, Dex responded as she'd hoped. His lips brushed hers, innocently at first, teasing. He tasted of chocolate and mint and hope.

This kiss was unlike the ones in the parking lot at the rest stop. This kiss held more than simple attraction. Lena projected her love for him into the embrace and hoped Dex could sense that she wanted, no, needed more.

He eased back on the kiss, but kept her contained within the circle of his arms. "Do you think we can give this a real try? I'm game if you are."

# CHAPTER THIRTEEN

As they entered the church, Dex waited for the dread that he'd been sure would come when he walked through that vestibule, but it never came. The last time he'd been in this sanctuary, he'd been left at the altar. The grin that spread across his face was from the realization that being here didn't hurt.

"It's about time the two of you showed up. I was thinking I might have to send a scout out and make sure you were alive," his mom called out. She glared down at them from above, perched on the top of a ladder where she was wrapping a string of lights around one of the stained-glass windows.

Dex glanced down at his watch. "It's only nine, Mama. You act like we rolled in at noon. Should you be up on a ladder? Maybe I should do that."

"We've got two locations to decorate. Mary and I have been here for ages already, unlike some of you lazy bones who couldn't be bothered to roll out of the bed until the sun had been up for hours." The Southern accent came out stronger with the censure in her tone. Jabbing a finger toward the opposite side of the church, she directed, "There are bows to go on the ends of each pew in a box over there. You two start with getting those put up. And don't give me any sass about being on a ladder, I know my own limitations."

"Yes, ma'am," Dex and Lena echoed. Their eyes met and they shared a small laugh. Today wouldn't be the day to test his mom's patience, and he was glad Lena seemed to be picking up on that.

The interior of the church was warm, so they shed their coats and scarves and tossed them onto the last pew. Dex guided Lena over to the overflowing box of red bows his mom had indicated.

While Lena pulled one of the bows from the box, Dex wrapped his arms around her from behind. "I'm sure I'll be as good at this as I was wrapping presents."

Leaning against his chest, Lena sighed. "You were so bad at that."

"At least we get to spend the day together."

She snickered and waved a hand toward his

mom and Mary. "With a pair of sixty-year-old women as our chaperones."

No sooner than the words were out of Lena's mouth, his mom barked out an order for them to hang the bows. He muttered under his breath, "You heard the general, hang the bows."

He took a step back from Lena and snatched one of the bows out of the box. They hung several without speaking, but that didn't mean they weren't saying anything. As each bow came out of the box, his hands brushed against hers. Their eyes met and lingered on each other as each bow was placed. With each graze of their hands, Dex wanted to clasp his fingers with hers and find somewhere private to see where those teasing touches might lead. Sharing a bed the night before without taking things beyond a few kisses had been akin to torture, but he was determined to do things right with Lena. She wanted to take the physical side of things slow, and he would honor that. But each touch of their skin, each kiss, made that harder.

When Tommy and Jill came in a little while later, they brought with them an excitement that filled the church. The smiles on both of their faces energized Dex, and he found himself humming a Christmas carol.

"What's this? Ebenezer Scrooge actually knows Christmas music? I am shocked." Lena poked him, grabbing a bow and hurrying to the other end of the pew.

He grinned and grabbed a bow before following her. "I know a lot of Christmas music, actually."

Tommy strolled over, still smiling broadly. "So, the way I hear it, the two of you had quite the romantic evening last night. Even went up to the High Bridge? You aren't trying to steal my thunder, are you, big brother?"

Dex grinned at him. He took Lena's left hand in his and brought it up to his lips just to tease his brother. "So what if I am?"

He considered—briefly—allowing the misunderstanding to continue, but he didn't want to scare Lena. It was less than twenty-four hours ago that they'd move out of the fake zone and into reality. From the moment he'd taken her hand and led her out onto the High Bridge, he'd known that one day he would be proposing to her, though. It just wasn't that time yet, but before he could correct his brother, Jill squealed and ran over.

On the eve of her wedding, she was even more bubbly and bouncy than usual. He'd have never guessed it was possible for her to get more excitable, but he'd just been proven wrong.

"Oh, my God, did you really propose to her last night? Tommy said you wouldn't, but I told him that you wouldn't have brought Lena home with you unless you were dead serious about her."

The excitement on Jill's face was overwhelming. Dex swallowed hard at the onslaught of energy coming his way. Her words rushed over him and crashed into his mind. Knowing that one day he'd propose to Lena and having everyone think that was this day were miles apart. He'd just came to terms with the idea of another serious relationship and having a future with someone. It was starting to feel like commitment was crowding in far too quickly, like a flash flood rushing up over his heart.

His voice cracked when he spoke. "We haven't been dating that long yet, guys. This Christmas is all yours. We aren't engaged."

There was an awkwardness to Lena's laugh, but she backed him up with her own confirmation that they weren't ready for that step. "Yes, we are so not to that point yet."

Slipping an arm around her waist, he leaned

close and whispered, "I like that you said 'yet,' though."

"Why would you think we were engaged?" Lena asked, and he had to admit it was a very good question. He should have thought to ask that one himself, because he thought he'd quashed that line of thought from his family the previous morning.

Jill looked at them with a cat-that-got-the-canary grin. "I'm guessing that you haven't seen the photos that High Bridge put up on the tourism page we help your mom run, have you?"

Dex shook his head, forehead wrinkling as he considered her words. "No?" he finally ventured cautiously.

Jill pulled out her phone and tapped a few times before holding it out to him. Her smile was now ear to ear. "That was some kiss. They even tagged it with 'I think we just had another proposal. #perfectproposalspot.' So if you didn't propose last night, you really missed your opportunity, and you'll have to work extra hard to find a better one now."

Pink tinted Lena's cheeks as they viewed the photographic evidence of last evening's embrace together. She grabbed another bow and busied herself attaching it to the next pew. Clearly an avoidance tactic, he thought.

Not that he blamed her. He'd really like to change the topic himself, but Jill and Tommy seemed to want to press the issue. Probably because they were so deliriously happy with each other that they wanted to infect everyone within reach with the matrimony bug.

Personally, Dex thought the matrimony bug felt a bit like the start of a nasty stomach bug in that moment. His stomach churned with a nervous anxiety, and a deep desire to change the subject rose up from his core. "Drop it, please," he entreated. "Focus on decorating for your wedding."

Focus on anything but embarrassing Lena further...

Anything but marrying him off to the first woman he'd been serious about in years...

Anything at all.

He grabbed a bow out of the box and passed it to Lena. Looking back at Tommy and Jill, he asked, "Don't you have some decorations to put up, or are you just expecting us to do everything for you?"

After spending the day decorating both the church and the reception hall for Tommy and

Jill's wedding, Lena was ready for bed. Unfortunately, they still had several more hours of wedding-related activities to go. She was used to being on her feet all day, but Dex's mom had kept them going nonstop for hours. She'd followed behind, tweaking half the decorations they'd put up, obsessing over making everything absolutely perfect.

It was as heartwarming as it was frustrating. Lena couldn't imagine her own mother hanging a single item of decor. Micromanaging the wedding planner or interior decorator hired to do the job? Absolutely. But she'd never be hands-on like Ruth Henry had been.

"You ready to go get through this ugly Christmas sweater rehearsal dinner mess?" Dex asked, holding the car door open for her.

"I'm as ready as I'll ever be." She reached out and straightened his sweater. "That color looks as good on you as I thought it would."

"It will look better off."

"Shh…" Fighting against the blush she knew was rushing up her cheeks, Lena admonished him. "We are going to be late for this thing if we don't get inside soon. Put those thoughts right out of your mind."

He grumbled good-naturedly, but took her hand as she stepped out of the car. "My vote is still for skipping. We could leave a note saying we were heading back to Nashville to elope. They'd never even question it."

She rolled her eyes at him, trying her best to stick to that same joking tone. "After you spent the entire day arguing that we weren't engaged. Sure."

The thought of marrying him was far from distasteful, though. In fact, she could imagine a future where she and Dex were married. She could see them in a house in the suburbs of Nashville, a little boy, a little girl and a dog. They'd make trips to see his family regularly, so that their kids knew what a grandparent's love felt like. Having seen just how quickly they welcomed her into their loving arms, she had no doubts they'd move the world for their grandbabies. Being around Dex and his entire family had been easier than she'd thought possible. Actually, it felt really right. Being part of a real family was a novel experience for her, one she found herself deeply longing to hang on to, and the very last thing she wanted was to go back to her solitary existence in Nashville.

She was getting ahead of herself. She and Dex had shared a single date and she was imagining their children. Exhaling quickly, she pushed the thought of that imaginary future out of her head. "Should we go in?"

"Let's get it over with." He opened the door to the church and they stepped in out of the cold. From the looks of things, they were the last to arrive.

His mom made a quick motion to him to join them at the front of the church. Lena followed up the aisle more slowly and sat next to Dex's aunt Peggy.

Jill wore a simple veil with what Lena could only assume was a custom-designed ugly Christmas sweater that had the words Bride-to-Be knitted into the Christmas pattern. It was hideous, but Jill's radiance overcame the sweater's deficiency. The way the young bride stared at her groom-to-be, clad in a matching Husband-to-Be sweater, sent a pang of longing through Lena's heart. She wanted what Jill had—a Henry man standing at the altar next to her with a goofy grin on his face.

Shifting her glance to Dex, she found him staring back at her. He winked at her before turning his gaze back to the pretend ceremony in front of him. Even the obnoxious sweater couldn't detract from how handsome he looked.

As she sat waiting for the rehearsal part of

the evening to be over, she wondered, was this the church where Dex had been left at the altar? He had never said, but she reasoned that it was possible, even likely. She searched his face for signs of upset, but all she could detect was happiness as he watched his brother and future sister-in-law practice their ceremony.

Soon, the rehearsal was done and they moved to a large room at the back of the church for the ugly sweater part of the evening. At the back of the room stood a table loaded down with finger foods and appetizers.

Lena's stomach rumbled at the sight. Lunch had been so long ago. She and Dex made their way over to the food and filled their plates quickly. They took a seat at one of the round tables placed along one side of the room. After getting something in her stomach, she let her eyes scan the room. She'd expected a small party, given that the wedding was tomorrow, but there was actually quite a crowd.

Suddenly, Lena stood. Her heart jerked as her eyes and brain tried to process what she was seeing. *Who* she was seeing. Blinking hard, she tried to clear what had to be a hallucination from her mind. There was no way that her lying, cheating ex-boyfriend could be standing in front of her. The man turned and she swallowed hard when she realized it wasn't Connor. Of course, it wouldn't be Connor. Why would he be in Westfield, Tennessee, of all places?

"Lena?" The concern in Dex's voice brought her back to a state of calm. "You look like you've seen a ghost."

"I thought I saw someone I recognized and had a momentary panic. I'm okay now." She waved vaguely at the man talking to Tommy. Now that she got a better look at the man, she could see he only bore a faint resemblance to Connor and not nearly enough that she should have panicked. "I am going to step out and get a little air, though."

"I'll come with you," he offered.

"No." She laid a hand on his forearm. "You are needed here. And I'll only be a moment."

Leaving him standing alone, Lena grabbed her coat and stepped out into the crispness of the winter night. Though the frigid air pained her lungs, she inhaled deeply several times. Looking up, she focused on the constellations shining bright in the clear, dark sky.

"What am I doing?" she said aloud.

"Hiding out to avoid giving me a real answer, if I had to guess." Dex's voice came from behind her.

Spinning to face him, she grimaced. "That could be at least partially true."

"I'm a good listener though, I promise. And whatever it is, we can talk about it. We can get through it." With a gentle hand, he brushed his thumb along the edge of her lower lip. "And if it's about Jessie, you don't need to worry about her."

"It's nothing. Completely stupid."

"Your reaction said that it was something." His eyes searched her face. "Every drop of color left your face."

Breath puffing out visibly in the cold, Lena closed her eyes for a moment. "I thought I saw Connor."

"Your ex?"

"Yeah." Looking up at him, she shrugged. "It's completely irrational. He'd have no reason to be here, and yet I thought I saw him."

There was a harshness to his inhale, noticeable in the quiet. "You looked afraid. Did he hurt you?"

"Not physically." She shook her head and moved away from his touch. Staring out at the sky, she continued, "But yes, he hurt me. He was the first man I ever said 'I love you' to. And I found out too late that he'd been playing me from day one."

"Ouch."

"Yeah. He only wanted me because of who my father is. He wanted to be department head. Looking back, I ignored a lot of warning signs. The tan lines where he'd had a wedding ring, the nights when he ignored my calls, the way he never wanted me at his place and insisted on coming to mine."

"He was married." Dex's words weren't a question.

"Yeah. Oh, he told me he was separated and in the process of getting a divorce. And then weeks after my father promoted him to head of Cardio, he and his wife decided to work things out. Later, I found out they'd never actually been separated and she had encouraged him to pursue a relationship with me so that he could get in good with the medical director."

"Your father?"

"Got it in one. Connor's actions told me who he truly was, but I didn't want to see the truth because I had fallen hard for him. Or at least I thought I had."

"Thought?" Dex moved toward her quickly, his gaze intense.

Her lips turned up in a hint of a smile. "My heart's been telling me a little something different lately."

"I know exactly what you mean." His arms circled her waist and pulled her into his chest. "It's crazy, isn't it, that we could find something so strong in such a short time?"

"Mmm…" With her arms wrapped around his neck, she tiptoed up. "Are you going to kiss me or not, Doc?"

"Definitely going to kiss you, Nurse," he murmured against her lips.

Every kiss with Dex became this magical experience. Undeniably fierce, yet layered with an unexpected tenderness. Comforting, when she let her guard down enough to let him in.

And every moment, every kiss, she trusted the man who held her a little more.

# CHAPTER FOURTEEN

DEX TOOK HER hand in his as they entered the church and he seated her with his aunt before leaving to find his brother. As best man, he couldn't stay in the sanctuary with Lena, even if she'd have vastly preferred that. So she settled in next to Peggy and they made a little small talk while they waited for the ceremony to begin.

Most of the guests were already inside and seated when Tommy came in and took his place at the altar. A goofy love-struck grin screamed to the entire church just how happy he was in that moment.

Dex followed right behind him. The matching grin on Dex's face warmed Lena's heart. The candlelight glow and remnants of sunset streaming in through the stained glass created this moody, intense lighting that highlighted all of his best features. Clad in dark reds and pine greens, the wedding party gathered at the front of the church to await the moment when Tommy and Jill would exchange their vows.

Crisp garlands of flowers mixed with shiny ribbons and ornamented wreaths. At the back of the altar, a large Christmas tree rose tall just beneath the cross. Christmas had never looked more romantic.

Lena struggled through the ceremony to keep her focus on the bride and groom. Even as Jill made her way up the aisle, as lovely as she was, her gaze kept drifting over to Dex. And given how often their eyes met, she knew he shared her struggles. As the pastor started the ceremony and even through the vows, Dex kept sneaking peeks at Lena.

He even missed the cue to pass Tommy the rings and had to be prompted.

"Looks like our best man has been distracted by that lovely young lady in the second pew," the pastor said with a teasing tone. The man's words sent a wave of tittering laughter through the church.

Lena's cheeks heated but she couldn't control the smile on her face. It took all the self-control she possessed to avoid rushing up there and throwing herself into his arms.

Peggy nudged her and whispered, "I do think that boy is in love with you."

Her eyes darted back to Dex and their eyes met again. His smile widened and her heart swelled. In his expression, she found hope. It radiated out and soothed the wounds talking about Connor had left jagged. It left her optimistic that the future would be bright.

"Relationships take love and they take work. Tommy, Jill, you've vowed to always love each other before all these witnesses, but it will also take commitment to stay dedicated to each other and to uphold what is best for your marriage." The pastor paused to allow the impact of the moment to build. "With that said, this is the moment where I have to ask those who have joined us here today for this momentous occasion to also make a promise—a promise to stand by this couple, to remind them of their vows if necessary, and to set the example of what love is and what family is. If you agree to this promise, please now confirm with your own 'I do.'"

The entire crowd yelled out, "I do."

Holding up a hand, the pastor waited for the sanctuary to grow quiet again. Finally, the last of the stragglers stopped chorusing their agreements and silence filled the church.

"Tommy and Jill, this room is filled with people who have pledged their support to you.

You will be starting your marriage strong and—"

He was interrupted by the sound of the sanctuary doors slamming open.

"Oh, I'm so sorry to interrupt! Don't mind me. I'll just find a seat." In walked a tall woman in a dress that was more appropriate for a night out at a club than a church wedding. Her long hair was styled in big curls that bounced around her as she strode forward on stiletto heels. She walked up the aisle like she owned the place, her steps sure and confident. Instead of taking a seat, though, she stepped up to Jill and hugged her tight. "Sorry, Jilly! I didn't mean to interrupt, really."

Lena knew without anyone saying that this was Jessie—the runaway bride, Dex's ex-fiancée. That thought was confirmed when the other woman blew a kiss to Dex.

"Hey, Dex. Maybe we can catch up after?" Jessie sashayed down to sit next to her parents, exaggerating her movements and keeping her eyes on Dex.

Dex had this totally gobsmacked expression on his face that Lena couldn't quite decipher. His gaze kept drifting over to where Jessie sat, the hem of her bright red dress creeping higher on her thighs.

Maybe it had been inevitable, but Lena had really hoped they could avoid Jessie. The way the other woman had looked at Dex, though, the desire and want shining brightly in her eyes, oh, her intentions were crystal clear. Jessie had realized what she'd lost and planned to rectify that mistake, no matter who she trampled in the process. A trickle of fear shimmied down Lena's spine.

Her heart hurt at the realization that once Jessie walked in, Dex had hardly spared her a glance. As Dex's first love, Jessie had a power over him that Lena did not. With their relationship being so very new, Lena wasn't sure that what they had was strong enough to withstand Jessie wanting him back.

The pastor came out of his shocked stupor and finished the ceremony, finally pronouncing Tommy and Jill as man and wife.

After the ceremony, Dex had to walk the bridesmaid out and stand for pictures. It looked like it might be some time before Lena would be able to reconnect with him. A little while longer before she found out once and for all where things stood between them. He sent her a quick wave and mouthed an apology.

When Jill grabbed Jessie and pulled her in for pictures, it sent another jab of panic running down Lena's spine. Jessie laid her head over on Dex's shoulder for one of the photos and they looked like a couple. Knowing that continuing to watch Jessie make a play for Dex was only torturing herself, Lena sighed and stepped away.

She made her way over to the reception alone.

"I finally escaped from that photographer. I think Tommy and Jill will grow old together getting their wedding photos taken." He kissed his aunt Peggy on the cheek. "Have you seen Lena?"

He needed to reassure her that seeing Jessie changed nothing for him. The stricken look on Lena's face when she had realized just who had made such a dramatic entrance to the wedding was seared into his brain. He had to make sure she knew how he felt before Jessie somehow made things worse.

For a horrible moment, Dex could imagine just what Lena had looked like when the truth about Connor had surfaced. Lost and vulnerable, she'd looked like she was seeing her world implode before her very eyes. He'd wanted to pull her into his arms, close that physical distance, and kiss her until they had to break for air or suffocate. The desire to do just that had been palpable, but he'd had to dismiss it. Jessie had already interrupted Tommy and Jill's wedding enough. He'd had to avoid looking at her for the remainder of the ceremony because if he'd seen even a hint of tears, he couldn't have remained standing next to his brother.

"Dexter, that young woman of yours is remarkable," his aunt Peggy said. "I do hope you know that you've found a keeper this time and don't let that painted-up tart ruin this for you like she nearly did Tommy's wedding."

"I hear you, Aunt Peggy. But first I need to find Lena."

Blowing kisses at him in front of an entire church full of people? Jessie couldn't have been more obvious if she'd hung a sign around her neck that said Property of Dexter Henry. After all this time, just when he was finally happy again, Jessie had to pull this crap. Why now? Was it just another way of torturing him?

"They are going to start dancing soon. You should go find your girl, because you two lovebirds don't want to miss out on that." Peggy jabbed his arm. "I hear rumors that destination weddings are what's going to be in style for next year. White dress, white sand, sounds like what's right to me, don't you?"

"Hint heard and noted."

"This one's worth fighting for. Don't you let her walk away." She winked at him before disappearing into the crowd. She wobbled slightly before righting herself. He considered that before continuing his search for Lena.

When his little brother entered the room with his new bride, Dex paused his search for Lena momentarily and joined in the applause that spread throughout the room. Tommy and Jill held hands, both smiling like lunatics, as they made their way to the head table. When Tommy kissed her before they sat down, someone cheered.

"We want to thank you all for being here to share this day with us. It means the world to us," Jill said. "Now let's dance!"

He scanned the crowd, looking for Lena. Their eyes met from across the room. He took one step toward her and someone screamed.

"Dexter!" his dad shouted.

Moving away from Lena with regret, he headed in the direction his dad's voice had come from. The crowd on the dance floor parted to let him through. His aunt Peggy lay sprawled out next to a chair along the edge of the room.

"What happened?" he asked, already reaching for her throat to take her pulse. Her heart rate was rapid and felt irregular under his fingers.

His dad looked on anxiously. "We were walking toward the dance floor and she said 'Oh, I think my blood sugar's crashing.' She walked away and fell before she got to the table."

"I should have followed up when I realized she was unsteady on her feet," Dexter said. "I should have read the signs."

Lena had hurried over from the opposite direction. She pulled a glucose monitor out of Peggy's purse and was checking her numbers already. The machine beeped and flashed a number that was far too low.

"She's had a hypoglycemic crash." Lena pulled an autoinjector syringe out of the purse. "Glucagon. She must be prone to this sort of thing."

"She's never passed out before that I know of." Dex's dad paced around next to them. The entire crowd was focused on them.

"You can't give her that. We don't know she needs it."

"This wasn't in her purse for no reason," Lena argued. "She needs it, and I'm giving it to her now." She pulled Peggy's sleeve up and pushed the autoinjector against her skin. Dex watched as she pushed the button and the clear liquid in the pen was dispensed into his aunt's arm. "We should roll her onto her side. This can sometimes cause vomiting."

"Has anyone called 911?" Dex asked as he rolled his aunt over.

"She also has glucose tablets and hard candies in her purse. I'm guessing her glucose plummets frequently." Lena put the purse down next to him. "She should wake up within a few minutes once this kicks in. I'm going to get her some food. Keep an eye on her."

Lena disappeared from his sight.

He brushed Peggy's hair away from her face and checked her pulse again. It was stronger and not quite as fast as earlier.

Swallowing hard, he couldn't help but be grateful that Lena was with him. He'd done rotations in general medicine, of course, but his knowledge of hypoglycemia was limited to it being a potential postsurgical complication that the nurses dealt with. Lena would have vastly more experience with this condition than he did.

Peggy started to stir. She muttered something incoherent and tried to sit up.

"Shh. We got you, Aunt Peggy." Reassurances slipped from his tongue. He helped ease her into a seated position. "Try not to move too much."

Lena came back with a small plate and a cup of soda. "Hey, Peggy. You think you could sip at this soda for me? I've got some of those tiny sandwiches for you too once you feel up to that."

Peggy's hand was shaky as she reached for the soda, but she managed to get it to her lips without spilling. After a few sips, she set it down and took one of the little sandwiches.

Paramedics came in then.

"Oh, you didn't have to call them. I'm fine," Peggy argued in a weak voice.

"You were unconscious. Yes, we did," Dex countered. Stubbornness ran in his family. She was not going to give in easily, that's for sure. He took a step back to give the paramedics a little breathing room.

Just as he turned to look for Lena, Jessie ran into his chest. Her arms snaked up around his neck.

"Oh, Dexter, I was so scared. You saved her. You actually saved her!" Jessie gushed. "My hero!"

Opening his mouth to argue that actually Lena deserved that credit, he froze when Jessie's mouth pressed against his and her tongue slipped past his parted lips. He struggled to comprehend exactly what was happening.

He put his hands on her hips and pushed her back away from him.

"Jessie, please don't do that again." Extracting himself from her clutches felt like trying to get away from the world's clingiest octopus. "What were you thinking?"

"I screwed up before, baby. You are my past, my present and my future."

Jessie really hadn't changed, though. After the time and the distance between them, he could see what a self-centered person she was. She still needed to be the center of attention, no matter who she hurt in the process. She'd never been anyone that he could have had a real marriage and a real future with. That was a lesson that had been driven home like a hammer pounding a nail into his thick skull. He'd left their wedding alone, his heart hollow and empty. And it wasn't until Lena came into his life, pelting him with shiny balls of ribbon, that he'd even realized how much he'd isolated his heart.

The carefree playboy persona he'd adopted after Jessie's betrayal had been scattered into the crisp winter wind after that mind-altering kiss he shared with Lena at the rest stop. Or maybe even before then. He couldn't be sure.

A few things he was sure of. One was that he'd never go back to Jessie. Two, quick hook-ups with no feelings would never be enough for him again. And most important, if he couldn't be with Lena, then he'd rather be alone.

He stepped back and she followed.

"Jessie, stop. You and I…never going to happen. Not again. I'm with Lena now."

Jessie flipped her hair over her shoulder, a sign he recognized as her doubling down on her efforts. He'd seen that exact motion many times during the years they were together. "I refuse to accept that."

"You'd better learn to accept it. Jessie, you are my past. And, honestly, you leaving me at the altar was the best thing that you've ever done for me. If it hadn't been for that, I'd have never ended up where I did, and I'd have never found Lena—the woman I intend to spend my future with."

Smirking at him, Jessie waved a hand. "You mean the girl who ran off when I kissed you. Some future."

*Ran off?*

He scanned the room. No sign of Lena.

His heart started racing. Jessie had ruined

him in this very church once. Had she done it again? He had to find Lena, fast, before it was too late.

Lena watched as Jessie threw herself into Dex's arms. As they kissed, her heart shattered into a million pieces. When Dex's hands moved to Jessie's waist, she couldn't bear to watch.

She left the reception and found herself in the sanctuary. In a town like Westfield, she couldn't just call an Uber. Especially not on Christmas Eve.

Maybe Wade could be persuaded to get her out of town.

She sank down behind the Christmas tree, wanting a little privacy for the breakdown that seemed inevitable at the moment. Tears lurked just behind her lashes, waiting impatiently for her to lower her guard and allow them the freedom to roll down her cheeks.

Dex had chosen Jessie. Just like Connor had chosen his wife. What was it about her that made men only want her when she had something to offer them?

For Connor, a promotion.

For Dex, a way to avoid matchmaking and potentially a way to make his ex-fiancée jealous.

She swallowed hard and wrapped her arms

around her knees. She'd trusted Dex too. Let him in, like she'd sworn she'd never do again. Little by little, he'd broken through the layers of ice around her heart and warmed her clear down to her soul.

And while she'd cared about Connor, and the end of their relationship had destroyed her, it never hurt this much. Seeing Dex kiss Jessie had felt like her heart and lungs had been ripped violently from her chest.

Gasping for air, she tried to remember how to breathe. This was what true heartbreak felt like.

"Lena?" Dex called from somewhere at the back of the sanctuary.

Sinking lower, she made herself small, hoping to avoid seeing him. How could she face him now? Knowing he had just been kissing Jessie after claiming to be all in with her?

She couldn't bear to look at him.

"Lena?" He called again from much closer. "Where are you?"

The door to the sanctuary banged open again, the sound of music growing louder until the door swung back closed. Lena breathed a sigh of relief.

"Dex, why are you in here alone when we could be dancing?"

Lena stiffened. She wasn't alone after all.

"Go away, Jessie." Agitation made Dex's voice rougher than usual. "I'm looking for my girlfriend."

"I'm standing right here, baby."

"Not you."

Lena peered through the tree at the hostility she heard from Dex. He was standing a few feet away, glaring at Jessie.

"But—"

"No *but*s. No *if*s. No us. Jessie, you left me standing at that altar in a tux. You disappeared without a word and didn't resurface for years. Surely you didn't think you could just come back and we'd pick up like nothing had ever happened?"

Lena watched as Jessie shrank back from his vehement tone.

"I hoped—"

"No." Dex ran his hands through his hair. "I love her. Don't you see? I am in love with Lena. And you might have screwed that up. Can't you just let me be happy?"

Lena's heart raced. *Dex loves me?*

A wisp of hope hummed through her, rising and thickening as she watched Dex crush Jessie's reconciliation plans. She choked back a sob, stuffing her fist to her mouth to muffle the sound.

But it was too late. Dex had heard.

He came around the tree, sank down next to her, and pulled her into his arms. "Lena, you have to know, you are the only woman I want. Getting back with Jessie has never once been a consideration for me."

"I'm standing right here," Jessie whined from the other side of the tree.

"And you can feel free to leave any time unless you want to hear me professing my love to another woman." Dex looked at Lena and rolled his eyes. "She never has been good at taking a hint."

Jessie huffed loudly and stomped out of the sanctuary.

When the door closed behind her, Dex sighed. "Okay, so, elephant in the room. I know you saw her kiss me. I didn't kiss her back. Admittedly, I didn't stop her immediately, but I panicked. My brain couldn't seem to process what was happening or how to make it stop."

"I saw tongue."

"Hers!" he insisted. "I swear. Honestly, that was what seemed to jar me back into action. It was only once I'd managed to detach her—

have I mentioned she's a major clinger?—that I could see you had left."

Her heart wanted to believe him.

"I won't be the other woman again."

"You've been the only woman I've looked at for months. Don't you know that?" Snorting, Dex squeezed her tight. "Since the day I asked you out and you shot me down so hard, you have been making me crazy."

"I don't believe that."

"Believe it." He captured her lips in a fiery kiss. Cupping the back of her head with one large hand, he held her as his lips roamed over hers and his tongue coaxed her lips to open. When it dawned on her that they were in a church, she pushed him back.

"Dex…" she started.

"I need to say something. Will you just hear me out before you reject me?" He stood and held a hand out to her. "Please?"

"Okay," she agreed. Putting her hand in his, she let him help her up off the floor.

Leading her around the tree, he stopped in the spot where his brother had stood earlier that evening. "A few long years ago, I stood right here in this very church and waited for someone who never showed. A few short weeks ago,

I just wanted to get in and out of this church with some of my pride intact."

"Where are you going with this?"

"Shh… Let me finish." He took a step back. "A few hours ago, I stood right here looking at you and realized that I wanted to be the groom. I wanted to be someone's husband. Your husband." He dropped to one knee in front of her. "I don't have a ring. I don't have some elaborate proposal planned. But I love you. Will you marry me?"

# CHAPTER FIFTEEN

*One week later*

THE FIRE CRACKLED brightly as Dex put another log on the flames. "Now, this is my idea of how New Year's Eve should be spent," he said as he walked back over to the couch and pulled the blanket back up over himself. "Just me and the love of my life, tucked away in a honeymoon cabin nestled in the Smoky Mountains."

They were only a few miles from his parents' house in Westfield, but this single-bedroom cabin afforded them the privacy that a newly engaged couple desired. They'd spent most of the week between Tommy's wedding and New Year's Eve with his family. Instead of staying for the party his family had planned, they'd decided to end the year snuggled up in front of a fire, just the two of them.

Lena placed her hand on his chest. She admired the way the shiny diamond Dex had slid on her finger on Christmas morning sparkled in the firelight. "I think when we do get married we should come back here. This place is perfect. I've never been happier than when I'm here with you."

"I haven't upheld my end of the bargain though. You met my family, dealt with all the drama with my ex, and we skipped out on going to LA for the gala to come here instead." He pressed a kiss to her temple. "I feel a little guilty about that."

"You have nothing to feel guilty about." She ran a single finger along his jaw. "It was my decision not to go to California and subject you to the scrutiny of my parents."

He shrugged. "I have to meet them someday."

"Why?" She saw no reason to force him to meet parents who had never put her best interests at heart. "You actually deserve the credit for the decision. If you didn't love me so much, and hadn't taken me home to show me what a real family looks like, I would never have known just how bad my family dynamic really was. You gave me the confidence—no, that's not the right word—the *courage* to stand up to them and refuse to accept their treatment of me any longer."

"You deserve so much better than that."

Dex gave her a newfound respect for herself that she hadn't known possible. For years, Lena had only been sure of herself when clad in scrubs and within the walls of a hospital. Outside, she was a different person, and when with her parents, she was even less than that. Her family's constant scrutiny and relentless inquisition made her a shell of a person.

But with Dex's love, she felt strong. Like she could face anything, and even stand up to her parents. She'd called them and told them she was engaged and while they were still screaming about that fact, she'd informed them that she was not only not attending the gala, but that she wasn't moving back to California either.

"And I found something...someone better."

Dex cupped the nape of her neck, which felt just right. The gentleness of his touch sent a warm tingly feeling down her spine. "Have I told you how much I love you?"

"I don't mind hearing it again."

If they lived to be one hundred and he told her one thousand times a day, it would never be enough. His lips brushed hers in the lightest ghost of a kiss. Her heart beat faster at the feel of being in his arms. Like breathing, she needed him close. His kiss fed her soul like oxygen fed her lungs.

"It's hard sometimes for me to believe how much my life has changed in less than a year."

He tickled her side. "Try less than a month."

"You're right about that." She laughed. "And to think, I almost didn't agree to your initial proposal. If I hadn't agreed to be your fake girlfriend, I'd have never become your real fiancée."

That was a truth that she hadn't managed to wrap her head around yet. She'd been so close to passing on an amazing man simply because she'd been scared. It was a hard thought to accept that she might have missed out on all this because of fear.

A slow, easy smile lit his face and brightened his face like the fireplace brightened the room. "Imagine how things would have turned out if I'd brought Belinda home as my fake girlfriend instead. I could have been engaged to a woman who came to the relationship not just with kids, but grandkids as well. I could have been a grandfather. I gave that up for you."

Lena laughed. "Well, you're mine now. Belinda will have to find her own surgeon to marry."

"Is that right?" he asked, and his gaze dropped to her lips. "So, getting back to the idea of that wedding and honeymoon, when did you have in mind?"

* * * * *